"The prolific Eric Maisel has produced yet another wise and useful book for counselors and psychotherapists. The 'humane' approach to understanding and helping clients described in this book is essentially a non-medicalizing and non-pathologizing approach that puts respect for clients at the forefront where it should be. Practitioners of all theoretical persuasions should find this book enlightening and helpful."

James E. Maddux, PhD, university professor emeritus, Department of Psychology, senior scholar, Center for the Advancement of Well-Being, George Mason University, Fairfax, Virginia

"In *Humane Helping*, Eric Maisel gives practitioners and healers powerful and practical tools for helping their patients grow, evolve, and transform. Through rich case examples combined with his hallmark timeless wisdom, Eric teaches us to step outside of conventional diagnoses and appreciate the full humanity in the patients we treat, and in ourselves."

Anna Yusim, MD, psychiatrist and author of *Fulfilled: How the Science of Spirituality Can Help You Live a Happier, More Meaningful Life*

"In *Humane Helping*, Dr. Eric Maisel provides therapists with practical recipes for healing. He discusses ways in which current diagnostic or fix-it paradigms can act as barriers to healing. He then provides us with in depth advice about how to be a more human, grounded, and skilled helper. A useful guide for beginning and experienced therapists alike!"

Melanie Greenberg, PhD, author of *The Stress-Proof Brain* and *The Mindful Self-Express* blog

Humane Helping

Humane Helping is a comprehensive, practical guide that helps clinicians shift their practice from the mental disorder-and-chemical fix and expert-talk models to a more humane, helpful model that increases their ability to help clients meet life's challenges and reduce emotional distress. Chapters clearly explain the shortfalls of the current models and the advantages of Eric Maisel's model and include case studies, reflection questions, and actionable steps. Written for helping professionals in mental health as well as practitioners from fields such as coaching and nursing, *Humane Helping* challenges current practices and provides helpers with the tools they need to more compassionately, effectively, and honestly serve their clients.

Eric Maisel, PhD, is a retired licensed psychotherapist, creativity coach, and internationally respected expert in the field of mental health reform. He is the author of more than fifty books including *The Future of Mental Health*, *Rethinking Depression*, *Overcoming Your Difficult Family*, and *The Van Gogh Blues*. He reaches a large audience with his personal list, *Psychology Today* blog, print column for *Professional Artist* magazine, and weekly appearance in the *Fine Art America* newsletter.

Humane Helping

Focusing Less on Disorders and More on Life's Challenges

Eric Maisel

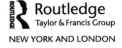

Routledge
Taylor & Francis Group

NEW YORK AND LONDON

First edition published 2018
by Routledge
711 Third Avenue, New York, NY 10017

and by Routledge
2 Park Square, Milton Park, Abingdon, Oxon, OX14 4RN

Routledge is an imprint of the Taylor & Francis Group, an informa business

Library of Congress Cataloging-in-Publication Data
Names: Maisel, Eric, 1947- author.
Title: Humane helping: focusing less on disorders and more on life's challenges / Eric Maisel.
Description: New York : Routledge, 2017. | Includes bibliographical references and index.
Identifiers : LCCN 2017023109 | ISBN 9781138038608 (hardcover : alk. paper) | ISBN 9781138038615 (pbk. : alk. paper) | ISBN 9781315115801 (e-book)
Subjects: | MESH: Mental Disorders—therapy | Professional-Patient Relations
Classification: LCC RC454 | NLM WM 400 | DDC 616.89—dc23
LC record available at https://lccn.loc.gov/2017023109

ISBN: 978-1-138-03860-8 (hbk)
ISBN: 978-1-138-03861-5 (pbk)
ISBN: 978-1-315-11580-1 (ebk)

Typeset in Sabon
by Keystroke, Neville Lodge, Tettenhall, Wolverhampton

For Ann, the epitome of a humane helper

Contents

Author's Note

I've conducted hundreds of print interviews with practitioners from around the world for my "Rethinking Mental Health" blog on *Psychology Today*. Throughout this book, I'll be saying that a given practitioner explained a point to me in an interview: in each case, I'm referring to an interview that appeared on my *Psychology Today* blog. Further references are included at each such juncture, in case you'd like to read the complete interview.[1]

NOTE

1 All interview excerpts have been reprinted with permission from *Psychology Today*.

Introduction

Help comes in all forms. Firefighters rush to save our houses from burning down, emergency medical technicians (EMTs) race to the scene of traffic accidents, and accountants help with our taxes. A teacher helps a first grader out of his raincoat, a lawyer helps his client stay silent when speaking would harm him, and a sommelier helps you select from among the hundred wines on the wine list. The ways in which human beings can be of help and are of help to each other are myriad and varied.

Who helps when you are in despair? Suddenly the picture gets very complicated. Is it actually the human-sounding thing called despair or is it the medical-sounding thing called "the mental disorder of depression"? Are we sad about life, did something break in our plumbing, or is it somehow both at once? If it is sadness, what sort of professional helper has anything useful to offer us, anything more useful than what a friend might provide us for free? If it is genuinely a "medical condition," why just talk about it with a helper whose practice centers around talk? Would you just talk about cancer or diabetes? This starts to look very murky indeed.

If the thing you are experiencing is despair, then part of the answer is that you must help yourself. Maybe you don't know how to put out fires and maybe you can't keep up on the tax code but we are obliged to learn how to help ourselves deal with our thoughts, feelings, moods, and circumstances. This sounds obvious and the thousands of self-help books available underline this idea. Yet there has appeared a burgeoning trend in recent decades that renames despair as the "mental disorder of depression" and announces to sufferers that they are afflicted by something that, in order to be eliminated, requires the equivalent of a firefighter or an accountant.

Because of this burgeoning trend, which is now the dominant paradigm of helping for virtually all problems of living that have an emotional component (like sadness), a behavioral component (like drinking too much alcohol), a personality component (like rubbing people the wrong way), a socially objectionable component (like being disruptive in class), or some other "negative" feature of human reality, people are primed to seek out a pseudo-medical solution. They may not know the technical differences among a psychiatrist, a clinical psychologist, or a psycho-therapist but they know that millions of people are taking pills for "conditions" of these sorts and maybe they (or their child or their loved one) should also.

In line with this burgeoning trend, helpers necessarily find themselves shifting away from a human-to-human model, the paradigmatic examples of which might be two friends chatting or a child talking with an aunt, to an expert-and-client or doctor-and-patient model where "mental disorders" are "diagnosed" and "treated," where "psychological tests" reveal "conditions" like an "attention deficit disorder" or a "personality disorder," and where "psychological issues" are taken out of the context of a person's circumstances and belief system and dissected as if they were specimens in a lab. Scientism and pseudo-science now regularly prevail.

We will look at these trends and discuss how you can sidestep them and practice as a humane helper. Helping another person who is suffering or whose behaviors are harming him or others is very hard, a truth we'll discuss in Chapter 1; but it is also easy, in the senses we'll chat about in Chapter 2. Whether it is hard or easy, if you have chosen helping as your profession you are obliged not to shy away from dealing with the person sitting across from you as if he were a human being and not a social problem or a medical patient. He may prove mysterious to you and you may find that you can only help him so much, but your starting point is a deep acceptance of your client's humanity.

Becoming a more humane helper is not beyond your reach. The operative word is "more," which mustn't be confused with "perfect." We sometimes do not even attempt to make a change, say in the direction of interacting more humanely with our clients, because we unconsciously set the bar at perfection. If we set the bar there we are likely to skip making any movement whatsoever in the direction of humane helping, since we know that perfection isn't attainable. But the options aren't "stay where I am" or "perfection."

A sensible, lovely option, and a great improvement over much of the help being currently offered, is "just a little more humanity, please." This might mean coming down from the high horse of "knowing" to the eye-level place of wondering and investigating, a subject we'll discuss in Chapter 3. It may mean refusing to cavalierly affix labels to your fellow human beings, a subject we'll discuss in Chapter 4, and also providing some wise counsel around the chemicals (called psychiatric medication) that your client may be desiring or may be receiving from another helper. It may mean training yourself to "hang out" with another person's emotionality rather than rushing to write a prescription, a subject we discuss in Chapters 5 and 6. All of these amount to more humane helping—and you can choose them.

Holding a rich, rounded picture of human nature, human reality, and the challenges of life is not that implausible a task. The main requirement is that you remember what life feels like to you, what sorts of odd messes and moods you've gotten yourself into, how "objectively" small slights have hurt you so much, the toll that year of hard drinking took on you, and so on. You keep a clear eye on your basic stance, that you are trying to help another human being, while actively disputing the two current dominant paradigms, the one of labels and chemicals that acts as if "everything is biological" and the second that reifies expert talk, turning ordinary helpers into "doctors of the mind." You opt for a third paradigm instead, the paradigm of humane helping.

Just by virtue of refusing to define people in terms of diagnoses and just by demanding of themselves that they remember how odd and complicated it is to be human, helpers, including mental health professionals, life coaches, and others, will automatically maintain a larger, broader view. They will refuse to reduce a person's reality to some set of psychological problems or putative symptoms of mental disorder and consistently exclaim, "Wow, being human is quite something, isn't it?" When helpers begin to do this honorable work, the helping professions will move in the direction of greater humanity.

In order to accomplish this shift in the direction of more humane helping, a helper must train herself to know about the current mental health system. She discerns the different players and their roles in the system, and how, in this odd landscape, one practitioner can be a Jungian analyst or a Freudian analyst and focus on dreams, another can prescribe pills, a third can administer psychological tests, a fourth can work exclusively on self-talk, and so on. Humane helping is essentially about your relationship with the person sitting across from you but it also requires an understanding of the current landscape of helping. A helper ought to be aware of the eye-popping implications of such a smorgasbord of approaches.

Likewise, a humane helper knows that there are a great many resources available to her clients that she may want to let them know about. She and her client aren't in a closed universe where only she can be of help and where her client is obliged to consider her his only source of help. It may strike her, for example, that the adolescent sitting across from her might be helped by a therapeutic wilderness experience, a mentoring relationship, a summer camp for creative youth, or peer counseling. If she believes this, she makes her beliefs known. That is the humane thing to do.

Likewise, our humane helper would advocate for a mental wellness movement that includes better conditions for everyone, less poverty, less hunger, less ignorance, less cruelty, more love—fewer of the bad things and more of the good things. She might pick a particular hobbyhorse to lobby for, such as teaching life skills in elementary school, teaching parenting skills to new immigrants, creating more communities of care, or supporting psychiatric survivor organizations. That is, she sees that a part of her role as humane helper is activism and that she is required to speak out and stand up.

Humane helping means the following: Your client is a human being and you are a human being. You are both mysterious, complicated creatures embedded in a particular time and place. In this time and place certain paradigmatic ways of dealing with human beings, the "doctor of the brain" model (psychiatry) and the "doctor of the mind" model (psycho-therapy) limit a helper's ability to "hang out" with her client in a safe, human-sized space where those mysterious complications may reveal themselves and where a helper may prove to be of great help. In this book, I hope to paint a picture of how you can be of genuine help in a world currently defined by two paradigms by opting for and practicing the third paradigm of humane helping.

1 Helping Is Hard

You are a mental health professional (or becoming one) or maybe you are some other helping professional. Maybe you're a licensed psychologist, a psychiatrist, a family therapist, a clinical social worker, a mental health counselor, or licensed or certified in some other way. You might also be a coach, workshop leader, alternative practitioner, or other helping professional who deals in a psychologically minded way with the people you see. You are accustomed to seeing people in emotional pain and distress and attempting to help them relieve that pain and distress.

You are likely somewhat or very aware of our current dominant mental health paradigm, which describes "mental disorders" in a certain way and which tends to lead inexorably to a chemical fix. You are also likely very aware that this way of looking at human distress leaves a lot to be desired. But, because of your training, your licensing mandate, and the fact that the current paradigm *is* the paradigm, you probably find yourself at a bit of a loss—or even at a great loss—to distance yourself from that paradigm and help your clients in ways that you suspect might serve them better. You may feel quite stuck in a profession and a system that, in order to make itself look expert and so as to wrap itself without justification in the mantle of science, isn't sufficiently serving its clients.

In this book, I want to explain how you can shift in the direction of a different, more humane, humbler but more honest paradigm, one that likely will feel better to you and will seem truer to you than the dominant medical-model paradigm and the secondary "expert talk about psychological issues" paradigm. This third paradigm, humane helping, looks at your clients as human beings suffering from certain problems and challenges with living and not from pseudo-medical conditions known as "mental disorders" or "mental diseases" and not exclusively (or primarily) from "psychological issues."

A movement is needed in the direction of humane helping and away from the twin ideas that mental health helping should be essentially or exclusively biologically oriented and the equivalent of medicine or that it should be essentially or exclusively psychologically oriented, erected on the scaffolding of so-called psychological theory, and played out as a certain sort of expert talk called psychotherapy. How lovely if you had a blood test or a urine test and if this were actually medicine or if Freudian theory, Jungian theory, cognitive-behavioral theory, or the other psychological brands were actual theories! But this isn't medicine; and there are no substantiated theories.

Humane helping of the sort I'll describe does a better job of taking into account human nature, acknowledging how little is known about the specific linkages that produce distress, and including for consideration aspects of a sufferer's life that are currently minimized or avoided altogether, aspects like a client's current circumstances, sociocultural conditions, life purpose choices, meaning needs, and original personality. This movement away from prescription pads and labels, on the one hand, and the pretension of psychological science, on the other, and toward warmth, honesty, clarity, and increased helpfulness is the subject of this book.

If you're a working mental health professional, the shifts and changes I'll describe will aid you in moving in the direction of providing care that matches our updated understanding of what helps to reduce emotional suffering and mental distress. Some of these changes are relatively easy to accomplish (like double-checking to see what your license mandate actually is), some are not too troublesome (like routinely checking in on a client's life purpose choices and meaning needs), and some are rather more difficult (like letting go of "mental disease" thinking and changing your body language from expert leaning back to engaged helper leaning forward). All of them, however, are doable—and if you accomplish *any of them*, your ability to humanely help will increase dramatically.

Nonetheless, even with your commitment to humane helping and your heroic shifts away from the current flawed dominant paradigms, helping will still prove hard. That hardness is part of the very nature of the enterprise, the enterprise of understanding another human being and finding ways to help another human being gain useful insights, make needed changes, learn new skills, adopt new habits, and change his or her worldview. How could any of that possibly be easy? It isn't.

You probably became a helper—a psychologist, a family therapist, a psychiatrist, a mental health counselor, a life coach, a clinical social worker, or some other helper—because you wanted to be of help. No doubt you had many reasons for your choice—ego reasons, a desire for professional prestige, a good income—but one of them was almost certainly your desire to ease another person's suffering and to help people live better, happier, more fulfilling lives. Then, very quickly, you came up against many significant—and sometimes harsh—realities. Let me describe fifteen of them.

The first is that people are difficult and sometimes extremely difficult. They possess formed personalities that make them rather intractably themselves. They obsess about things, they have their stubborn ways of doing things, they harm themselves, they may not seem overly concerned about actually relieving their distress, and they may hold that they have no particular problem—rather, everyone else has the problem. Human beings aren't easy to fathom, deal with, or help; and your decision to humanely help your fellow human beings will push you squarely up against this reality.

The second challenge is that people—our clients, you and me, and everyone else—are rather surprisingly thin-skinned and defensive. We take as criticism or as insulting anything unflattering being pointed out to us and we charge you with some sort of disloyalty or betrayal when you offer up your honest appraisal of our situation. On television shows played for laughs, television shrinks can be as sarcastic and caustic as they like. In real life, you will not have clients if you are sarcastic and caustic and even opting for just some gentle truth-telling may cause waves. As a result, helpers tend to proceed diplomatically, with kid gloves on—which a client may receive as humane and supportive but which may leave a lot of truth out of the interaction.

Third, it isn't all that easy to discern what a sufferer actually wants or needs. He may come in already self-diagnosed and believe that he wants help with his attention deficit disorder (ADD), post-traumatic stress disorder (PTSD), or depression, using the labels of the dominant paradigm, and because he is presenting himself that way you may have a hard time getting at what's causing his distress. He may be reticent to reveal his secrets, embarrassed to disclose what's really on his mind, or not very practiced at investigating his thoughts, feelings, history, or circumstances. Furthermore cause and effect is often impossible to discern when it comes to human distress, given that an objectively small event in a person's life, like a piece of criticism he received thirty years ago, may still be producing large consequences today.

Fourth, even if you acquire a decent sense of what a client wants and needs—say, to heal from a particular past trauma—it isn't at all clear what tactics and strategies will help achieve the results you and he would like to see. How does one person help another person heal from trauma? How does one person help another live with a bully, relieve a lifetime of sadness, or calm a seriously anxious nature? How does one person help another person change his inner language, grow more confident, or change his circumstances? Yet a helper is supposed to be adept at achieving outcomes of this sort. Is this really so easy?

Fifth, helping is not just an in-session sort of thing where two people have a particular kind of conversation. For a client to actually be helped, he must go out and do things: turn an insight into a new habit, improve his parenting skills, produce self-talk that serves him better, employ an anxiety management strategy in a real-life situation, speak more confidently at home or at work, look at life differently, engage in new behaviors that align with his new intentions, and so on. A helper can't go out and do these things for her client. Her client must do them. And human beings are not so good at making these changes. So, a next session with a client may begin on a somber note, that not much has changed and that your client feels guilty, embarrassed, and defensive about that lack of change. Over time, not much progress may be made, frustrating client and helper alike.

Sixth, you have all of your own shadows to contend with, the way you sometimes get bored in session, the way that your client's emotionality may frighten you, the way that your own chattering brain may prevent you from staying present, the way that your need to look right and to quickly problem-solve may inhibit your ability to relax and be patient, the way that your desire to look professional and appear to be an expert may cause you to act as if you know much more than you actually know. Indeed, you may need your own humane help—you may be despairing, still not healed from trauma, overly anxious, rigid and controlling, or in other ways struggling or difficult. The long and the short of it is that you will almost certainly have to contend with you.

Seventh, your life experiences likely prepared you very little for this sort of helping. You may have grown up in a family where you were expected to excel and succeed, not be of help to others, and your experiences in helping may have been limited to helping with the dishes or the yard work. Nor were you asked to be of help in your school years, except of course that you were admonished to cooperate and sometimes subjected to group projects where any hint of helping was construed as bossiness. Even if you did acquire some actual experiences of helping, for example because you participated in a peer counseling program in your high school, those few experiences could not have really prepared you for a sullen family walking into your family therapy office. It is a hard fact that you are forced to learn how to help via your on-the-job experiences.

Eighth, your training almost certainly didn't prepare you to help. Each training program has its own emphasis, an emphasis that amounts to the primary focus of the program—some emphasize independent research that adds to the psychology literature, some emphasize learning how to administer psychological tests, some emphasize psychopharmacology, etc.—and virtually none focus on "what helps" or even spend much time on the idea of helping. Generally, it's in your internships that you learn how to actually help; training programs typically hand that important responsibility over to the placements they partner with, meaning that each student learns only what his or her placement has to teach. As a rule, training programs provide no systematic or intensive education on what one might suppose is their central mandate, training helpers in helping.

Ninth, what if the thing you are trying to help with is a core feature of your client's original personality? How do you help with something that a person fundamentally "is"? Say that your client was born with a ton of life energy and appetite. She has been squirming, moving, rushing, eating, drinking, grasping, and bursting with energy since birth. That is who she is. Over time, this basic energy may have caused her all sorts of difficulties—an inability to sit still in her college classes, a restlessness that has led to misadventures, bouts of over-drinking and over-eating, and so on—which, however, are not "features of a mental disorder" but direct results of her natural bursting energy. How is a helper to help with aspects of personality that are original to the person? This reality, that clients come into the world already somebody and already themselves, is generally ignored in training programs, completely left out of a helper's education, and likewise finds no place in the two dominant paradigms.

Tenth, you're likely obliged to deal with a whole professional apparatus, with its language, ideas, constraints, operating procedures, and so on, that may handcuff you a little or a lot in your helping efforts. You will have reporting obligations, report-writing obligations, "standard of care" obligations, and formidable proscriptions about a million things, from taking a small present from your client to hugging your client to even shaking hands with your client. How human does all that sound? Given that there are only so many hours in a day and that many of these professional tasks are tedious and onerous, a helper may feel genuinely taxed by these professional obligations.

Related to this challenge is the challenge you face as a private practitioner to function as an entrepreneur. You may have a bevy of advertising, promoting, and marketing tasks, the need to sublet your office for a portion of the week so as to make ends meet, the maintenance of a web presence, the need to be savvy about and stay on top of technological innovations (like appointment software), and the abiding challenge of bringing in enough clients and enough income. Shadow features of this need to make money might include the desire to hold on to clients and to make them feel guilty for wanting to leave; and sitting on insurance panels whether or not you believe in the "diagnosing and treating mental disorders" paradigm. If you are in private practice, helping clients is made harder by the fact that running a successful business is itself time-consuming and hard.

Eleventh, you must abide by your licensing mandate, if you are a licensed professional. The licensing laws of each state are idiosyncratic—and often internally contradictory. In one paragraph your licensing law may state that you are entitled to practice independently; and in another paragraph, it may assert that if your client displays the symptoms of "mental illness" that you are then obliged to refer your client to a psychiatrist or other medical doctor and enter into a working collaboration with that doctor. Would any helper be able to parse that distinction? These are the sorts of tortuous twists encountered in licensing language.

Are you obliged to "diagnose and treat mental disorders," are you somehow restricted to only handling "psychological problems," or do you have the latitude to frame your work as "dealing with the ordinary problems of living" and practice as more of a humane helper? You may discover that you have more freedom than you supposed to work humanely and eclectically and this knowledge may help motivate you to make the changes I'll be suggesting. On the other hand, you may discover that you are even more constrained than you had supposed, which will come as a splash of cold water in the face—and amount to a poignant, ongoing problem.

Twelfth is the nature of the medical-model paradigm that currently dominates the mental health landscape. In all places and times there are dominant ways of dealing with human phenomena, whether that phenomenon is breaking the law, speaking truth to power, squirming in third grade, or despairing. That dominant way is called a paradigm: the agreed-upon way to view a thing. Right now, there exists a predominant paradigmatic way of viewing human phenomena as diverse as feeling sad, hearing voices, opposing your parents, or fearing snakes. That is the "mental disorder" paradigm.

This predominant paradigm asserts that when it comes to human suffering and many other human phenomena, there is an expert class that knows what's going on and what to do about it. These experts assert that "mental disorders" are real things (like elephants) and not imaginary things (like unicorns) or metaphors (like spring fever). A "mental disorder" is exactly like a "physical disorder" and shares the same reality, prestige, and tangibility as a "physical disorder." As hard as it may be to do so, our humane helper must make it her business to understand this paradigm, see what she thinks about it, and reject it (or certain parts of it) if she finds it untrustworthy and illegitimate.

This paradigm operates everywhere around you: as you watch television and find yourself bombarded by drug ads; as colleagues, peers, friends, and family members seriously discuss attention deficit hyperactivity disorder (ADHD), PTSD, clinical depression, bipolar disorder, obsessive-compulsive disorder, adult ADD, or some other "mental disorder" among themselves and with you, perhaps soliciting your advice, perhaps wondering what you think about a certain popular drug treatment; and in countless other ways, including in your dealings with health maintenance organizations (HMOs), in-patient facilities, social services, and the courts.

Thirteenth is what is likely your serious lack of knowledge about alternative resources and alternative paradigms (like humane helping) different from and in addition to the two dominant paradigms, the pseudo-medical "diagnosis and chemical fix" paradigm and the "expert talk" paradigm of psychotherapy. Our humane helper will make an effort to understand the alternative and competing paradigms available to her and make up her own mind about which feel most truthful and congenial to her and which best capture what she believes is the essence of genuine helping. For instance, she might investigate and then adopt a "human experience" paradigm that elevates "human experience" to the center of the helping picture, rather than marginalizing it or eliminating it from the picture. In that way, she could focus on "a client's life" rather than "a client's symptoms."

Fourteenth is burnout. If you've been helping for a long time, or even just for a few years, you may have figured out your ways of meeting or coming to terms with many of the above challenges and difficulties. You will have had many real life helping experiences that inform your helping style and you'll likely have figured out your way to live inside your license and deal with report-keeping, billing, reporting requirements, and so on. However, many of these challenges can never be completely resolved, including especially the intractability of human nature and our species' resistance to change. Because many of these challenges won't "go away," because you may grow seriously tired of having to tell yet another client that "we have to settle on some diagnosis just for insurance purposes," and because doing anything for a very long time can breed boredom and contempt, burnout may come to challenge you.

Fifteenth, because helping is really this hard and because clients may not want to change or really cooperate, a helper and her client may collude in taking it easy. A psychotherapist and his or her client might repeatedly discuss the same material, colluding in not pressing for change, since the client finds chatting easier than changing and the helper experiences this as an easy (if dull) and lucrative arrangement. A psychiatrist and his or her client might collude to agree that the client "has" some condition that requires a chemical fix. A Jungian analyst might start every session with, "And what did we dream about this week?" finding dream investigation enjoyable if not productive. This colluding may reduce the stress on both helper and client but over time may frustrate the helper because of its basic inauthenticity. That sense of inauthenticity then becomes its own challenge.

What do the above fifteen challenges suggest? That:

1. You will need to deal with the reality that people are difficult.

2. You will need to deal with the reality that people are defensive and hate feeling judged and criticized.

3. You will need to be easy with not knowing very much about what is "really" going on with or in your client.

4. You will need to be easy with not knowing for sure what works to relieve human suffering and distress, either generally or with respect to the person sitting across from you.

5. You will need to learn how to motivate your clients and exert positive influence, since helping is not just about what is said in session but about what your client actually accomplishes between sessions.

6. You will need to upgrade your personality, minimize your shadows, calm down, manifest your courage, not act exploitatively, and be your human best.

7. Because your experiences growing up and in school (perhaps including graduate school) probably provided you with very few genuine helping opportunities, you will need to supplement your life experiences with actual helping experiences.

8. Because your undergraduate and graduate program and/or your medical training probably did not emphasize helping enough, and maybe even avoided teaching helping, you will need to supplement your education and training with self-education and self-training.

9. You are obliged to deal with those features of human nature that "come with the creature," including whatever original endowments, proclivities, and preferences are built into the person sitting across from you.

10. You must contend with all of your professional obligations and the paraphernalia of professionalism, from reporting duties to report-keeping duties to running an office to maintaining your theoretical orientation (or shedding it in favor of a more humane eclecticism).

11. You are obliged to know what your license mandates that you do and not do; and if your licensing requirements prevent you from operating in ways that seem humane and sensible to you, you are likewise obliged to tackle that constraint, perhaps through activism or perhaps by retiring your license and working in a non-traditional way.

12. You need to understand the major shortcomings of the two dominant paradigms in the mental health field, the "diagnose and treat mental disorders" paradigm (that usually leads to a chemical fix) and the "expert talk" paradigm of psychotherapy, and how you intend to relate to them and deal with them.

13. Likewise you will want to understand what alternative paradigms are available to you, including those that do not invite or involve diagnosing, and what additional helping resources exist for people in distress, in addition to "expert talk" and a "chemical fix."

14. You will have to guard against the burnout that, since helping is hard, taxing on your system, and sometimes significantly frustrating, often accompanies years of helping.

15. You will need to keep an eye peeled for that internal pull to collude with your clients and act as if providing a label is the same as helping or that repeatedly talking about an issue is the same as progress and change.

All of these many realities are frustrating. It is certainly frustrating that people can be so difficult, stubborn, defensive, and intransigent, so unwilling to change or to make the requisite effort to help themselves, and so often self-sabotaging and quite often indifferent to relieving their own suffering. This is human nature—my nature, your nature, and your client's nature—and a bedrock difficulty that makes it hard for a helper to succeed at helping. In your naivety and idealism, you may have presumed that your clients would meet you at least halfway; and here they are, clinging to an addiction or to other behaviors that are harming them.

Your ability and your desire to humanely help your clients are negatively affected by the hardness of the task. But that doesn't render helping impossible. The hardness of the task should cause us to approach helping with some humility, rather than arrogant assurance, some energetic engagement, rather than practiced aloofness, and some measured optimism, too, because in the course of our helping we will see some—even many—of our clients change, heal, make progress, and enjoy life more. Humane helping is indubitably hard; but it may be exactly the sort of work that you find meaningful and that moves and inspires you.

POINTS FOR REFLECTION

1. In your mind, what do you take humane helping to mean?

2. Is humane helping a primary goal of yours or is it secondary to some other goal, like diagnosing and treating mental disorders, practicing psychotherapy, administering psychological tests, building a practice, achieving professional status, and so on?

3. Reflecting on the fifteen challenges described in this chapter, which seem the most intractable?

4. Reflecting on the fifteen challenges described in this chapter, which seem most pertinent to you?

5. Do you suspect that you'll find the hardness of the job of humane helping daunting or do you think that you will find ways to take that hardness in your stride?

2 Helping Is Easy

Humanely helping another human being is genuinely hard, for all the reasons we discussed in the last chapter. In the following senses, it is also easy. Here are ten significant reasons why helping is (or can be) easy.

1. THE EASE OF NOT TREATING AND NOT CURING

As a humane helper who has her doubts about the current "diagnose and provide chemicals" paradigm, you are not setting the bar at "cure" or even at "treat." You are simply trying to be of some help to the people you see. Your client is on a complicated, mysterious journey and his or her current distress, whose "causes" are likely unknown to him and likewise unknown to you, can't be "treated" like a rash or "cured" as if it were a disease.

This may not be what your client wants to hear or what your client thinks you ought to be offering. He may believe that you are indeed supposed to be "treating" him or "curing" him. You will need to disabuse clients of this notion by being clear that you hope to be of some help but that this isn't anything like a medical relationship. If you are clear in this regard, then you will have put your relationship on the right footing from the beginning and you will have made your job much easier.

If you see yourself as an expert who is diagnosing and treating mental disorders or who is a genuine "doctor of the mind," then you have created certain obligations that you can't really meet. But if you see yourself as trying to be of some help to a person experiencing distress or having problems meeting the challenges of living, that way of looking at what you are attempting to do underscores two patent realities: first, you may only be of some limited help and, second, this is your client's journey and not yours. While you may prove a "friend and helper along the way" you are not his surgeon or his salvation.

We expect our plumber to fix our pipes. But we do not expect our friend, however wise, experienced, sensitive, or compassionate she may be, to "fix" us. We expect her to listen; we expect that she may offer some suggestions; we expect that she may tell us a hard truth or two; we hope that she'll have some insight that proves useful and some ideas that we can act upon. But we don't expect her to "fix" us. As a humane helper, you come from this exact same place, which is different from, easier than, and more truthful than the "I am an expert with the tools to fix you" place.

2. THE EASE OF PLANTING SEEDS

A second place of ease has to do with results and outcomes. It is a place of genuine ease to recognize that the benefits your client receives from his time spent with you may not be yours to witness. You do not have to be upset, irritated, self-critical, or agitated if your client appears to make little or no progress during your time together. You may have planted some very important seeds that are destined to make a huge difference in his life. This is not a fanciful idea or a way to rationalize a lack of visible results. Rather, it happens all the time.

A gardener would not expect that the seed she just planted to sprout and flower the next day. As a humane helper, the same is true with respect to the helping work you do. You may say something to your client or your client may say something to you that doesn't register on first hearing or that he isn't prepared to act on now. Six months from now, however, that "long ago" interaction may allow him to enter into recovery, stop harming himself, make a change in his circumstances, or do something else really helpful. Yes, it took him that long; but it might never have happened but for the seed that was planted in your office.

This gardening analogy is apt. A significant portion of the work you do with clients involves helping them "cultivate" better habits and improved mindsets and it may take them some time to "own" these new habits and mindsets. Therefore, since seeing results isn't the only proof that something helpful and useful has transpired, you don't have to treat results as the absolute measure of whether or not you have been helpful. Seeing results is lovely; having your client thank you because he sees results is excellent; and your work together is *also* likely to bear fruit in the future. This makes helping easier.

3. THE EASE OF JUST BEING

By your very presence, if you are calm, interested, and present, you will help a bit with your client's existential agitation and loneliness. Helping is made easier simply by virtue of the fact that you are a human being, too, and an available one at that; and it may well be a bit of relatedness that your client needs the most at this moment.

As is often said, your client may already have all the answers she needs. But she may not be able to access those answers because she is currently too agitated or too morose. You, by your very being, by the way you smile and see her and relate to her, may provide the warmth, the calm, and the glimmers of hope that allow your client to speak her own answers. We'll chat more about this "simply being there" in subsequent chapters. Here I want to underline how fortunate it is that what a client may want and need the most, a present, sympathetic you, is also the easiest way for you to be, once you learn how to do it.

It is much harder to spend a day acting like an expert than just being a person. Imagine if you didn't have to stiffen your back, pull out your mental textbooks, justify the Diagnostic and Statistical Manual of Mental Disorders (DSM), and the logic of prescribing chemicals for an unhappy marriage or a terrible job, and in a hundred other ways seem to know things that you do not know and adopt models and paradigms that you do not respect? Imagine if you could just be, person to person, existing in a light, friendly, human place? Wouldn't that make helping much easier?

4. THE EASE THAT COMES BECAUSE YOU KNOW SOME THINGS

You can't be an expert in the same sense that a plumber or a surgeon can be an expert. You can't know another human being in those ways. We'll discuss this reality in the next chapter. But while that is abundantly true that isn't to say that you can't know things—even a lot of things.

You may know something very important about what can help an anxious client deal with his anxiety. You may know something very important about what can help a hopeless client regain hope. You may know something very important about what can help a despairing client change and improve his circumstances. You may know something very important about what can help a sullen teenager change his mind about acting out and failing at school. You may in fact know lots of things and possess an arsenal of tactics and strategies that you have tested in the crucible of the reality of your work with clients.

In this regard, you are very different from a "mere" friend. You are an experienced helper (or will become an experienced helper) who knows many things. Knowing the things that you know and possessing the strategies and tactics that you possess make helping easier. If, for example, you can teach an anxious client an anxiety management technique that is portable and that she can use in every situation where she finds herself anxious, that information will really serve her. And having that strategy to teach makes things easier on you, as you don't need to sit there not knowing what to do. You can say, "Let me teach you this little technique and let's see if it makes a difference in your life." That's the epitome of ease.

Likewise, because you are experienced, you don't have to jump on every issue that a client brings up as if it were "the" issue to be investigated and handled. Many times, you may have a practiced intuition that the "real" issue is coming but hasn't arrived yet. You can be helpful in the moment but also patient and easy as you await the next development, which, for example, may be your client saying, "You know, I think the truth of the matter is that I'm deeply lonely."

Nor do you need to jump on this news immediately, either, even if you think it is the "real" issue or a very important issue. First you would just "be there," so that your client has a chance to hear what she just said. Soon, however, you will be chatting in a territory that matters a lot to her, in this case the territory of loneliness. Getting there was easy because you didn't need to jump on every issue leading there and could let her (and help her) get to her destination without halting at all the whistle stops along the way.

With experience, you will know how to be there, how to listen, how to respond gently but firmly, how to make suggestions, how to wonder aloud about your worries about your client, how to conceptualize what's going on in tentative ways, how to game plan and how to change your game plan, and more. All of this knowing makes helping easier than if you didn't know. It may take you some time to acquire this knowing, which means that helping may feel harder at the beginning than as you gain more experience. But that is natural; and knowing that it may well get easier is itself a comfort.

5. THE EASE OF BEING WITH THE "HARDEST" FOLKS

Even those individuals deemed by society as the hardest to reach, the most troubled, the least responsive, the most traumatized, or in some other important sense the "hardest possible clients" may, because of your mindset and your practiced way of being, not prove so impossibly difficult to you. Consider the clinical social worker Roxanne Tonn, who works with chronically "mentally ill" and homeless individuals and helps them during their darkest and most difficult times. Her effectiveness with these populations has earned her a reputation as a "schizophrenia whisperer." She explained to me:[1]

> To be a humane helper means I must show up without judgment, without anxiety and with calm, fully present energy. If I am engaged in the moment, I have a chance to assist someone else. It gives space for the other person to "rest" in the calm energy that I am providing. Anxious energy, the idea of needing to fix someone, or that I have to solve "this" is disturbing to me and not productive to the person I am helping. It only agitates the already agitated. Pure calm energy will provide the space for real solutions to appear.
>
> I learned how to be a humane helper through my own experience as someone who supposedly needed "fixing." I never believed the labels I was given by people who barely knew me. I was born curious and I questioned everything in society that did not seem to be working. I questioned traditions and why people did what they did. I did not believe that being an explorer and cynic by nature should have instantly deemed me "crazy." My rebellious spirit and questioning of authority was not a disease to be medicated away; but society tried and told me that I would not succeed without chemicals.
>
> I went on to complete my master's in clinical social work without medications. I began my career working with the most severe population, dual-diagnosed homeless individuals. They are considered

the most "sick" by our society. They are the ones people run away from. I chose to run toward them because they are people too, regardless of the labels society puts on them. I knew that if I applied my humanity and understanding I could work with anyone. I was able to do that and became known as the "schizophrenia whisperer."

I was the person called when a client was incoherent or rambling uncontrollably. I sat with them person to person and put all labels aside. I made no judgments and worked without fear. This simple human interaction de-escalated the situation and made a difference with my clients. It was not the person that needed fixing, it was often the system they were trapped in. By adopting this approach people were no longer problems to be fixed but lives to be led.

It may not prove to be your job or your calling to work with the "most difficult" among us. But if you do work with them, or if you must work with them, you may find some real ease even there. No one knows for certain why folks in extreme states are experiencing what they are experiencing. You can't know either. The "system" may make pronouncements and act as if labeling someone "psychotic" and providing chemicals amounts to all the clarity necessary. However, you will know better and recognize that clarity has not been achieved by virtue of some chemical intervention. There is a kind of ease in this astute knowing.

6. THE EASE OF SMALL THINGS MATTERING

A small thing that you say to your client may matter a great deal to him. Indeed, your client may well tell you a session or two after the fact, "When you said that one thing to me two weeks ago, that made a real difference." The same with some small gesture—a smile, you leaning forward, or you cocking your head in thought. These may matter out of all proportion to the size of the gesture. Likewise, a small bit of advocacy may matter a lot: for example, providing your client with information about a certain resource after you said in session that you would.

Some small thing that you recommend may really matter. Maybe you recommend that he "think thoughts that serve him." You explain a bit about what you mean; you answer any questions he may have; together you identify a few thoughts that "aren't serving him"; you practice disputing them in session; together you come up with some thought substitutes that he can use when he finds himself thinking those unhelpful thoughts again. This is all basic cognitive work and really boils down to the suggestion that your client begins to "think thoughts that serve him." It takes no more than a few seconds to articulate the central message of cognitive therapy; and the positive results you obtain may be completely out of proportion to the small amount of time you spent describing this simple idea.

A simple remark, a small suggestion, an innocent gesture may all matter a great deal to the person sitting across from you. You do not have to struggle to be eloquent or to provide huge ideas and grand gestures. The accumulation of these small things, all these remarks, suggestions, and gestures, may lead to the grand result that clients feel better, harm themselves less, make wiser decisions, and experience less distress. You said a small thing while wearing a certain smile and that changed your client's life: how easy was that?

7. THE EASE OF PERMISSION

If what your client really needs to do is to say something out loud, this is a safe place for her to do that. This is the place where she can say that she feels ashamed, that she feels unloved, that she feels defeated, or that she feels worthless. Where else can she say such painful things? And isn't being able to say such painful things in a safe place a profound blessing?

It can feel easy to give clients this permission or it can feel scary. This may prove a place of growing ease for you because in the beginning you may feel consumed by the worry, "What am I supposed to do now?" It may feel anything but easy to hear your client's admissions as you fret about how you're supposed to react. Over time you will learn that there is nothing that you need to do, that your client is not hoping to be miraculously rescued by some brilliant thing that you say, that she doesn't need you to compliment her on her courage or acknowledge how hard it must have been for her to make that admission. What she needs is a certain kind of silence and a special holding of the moment.

This silence and this holding are actually easier than "doing something." You might even close your eyes for a moment, signifying that the two of you have come to "one of those places in life" that are the hardest, the most human, and also the most healing and liberating. You might close your eyes, breathe, and open your eyes—and there the two of you are; and your client may be transformed. It may be that she has needed for years, decades, or virtually forever to have said this. Now it is said; saying it didn't slay her; she is still alive; you haven't recoiled or vanished; and some ten-ton weight may have been miraculously lifted off her shoulders. And, for you, it was easy; you did the very best "nothing" possible.

8. THE EASE OF NOT STRIVING AND NOT ATTACHING

You want to help your clients and you hope that they will feel better because they worked with you. These desires, however, are not the same as striving for any particular results, especially "high bar" ones, or attaching to your clients in a clinging or needy way. If your client has been anxious her whole life, you would be setting the bar in an unreasonably high place if you said to yourself, "I will rid her of all her anxieties" or "With my help she will never be anxious again." To say such things means that you are holding some version of a "cure" mindset instead of the more appropriate "helping" mindset.

If you take it easy and do not strive for "high bar" results, you will do your most human work and you will also make helping that much easier on you. Likewise, you will make helping easier on you if you do not attach to your clients and if you do not hope too much that they succeed in some way, change in some way, or improve in some way. Nor should you cling to them because they are a source of income, because working with them makes you feel wanted, because working with them makes you seem like an expert, because working with them makes you feel powerful, or for any other shadowy reason having nothing to do with wanting to help them. Striving and attaching both make the work harder, tire you out unnecessarily, and are neither wanted nor appropriate.

9. THE EASE OF NOT BEING REVEALING

A humane helper is not obliged to be revealing. In fact, it is better on balance not to be personally revealing and not to share your stories, anecdotes, and experiences, not out of defensiveness but because sharing has a way of changing the energy in the work. We want to be authentic but authenticity does not come with the demand that we reveal ourselves.

It is a fortunate coincidence that not revealing is both better than revealing and also easier than revealing.

Some humane helpers like to use personal revelations as part of their way of working. This way of operating may make particular sense in certain settings, say in a peer counseling, mentoring, coaching, or twelve-step context. It may also make perfect sense as an occasional tactic in any helping setting and context. It might be good for an anxious client to hear how anxious you sometimes get or for an addicted client to hear how seriously long it took you to quit smoking cigarettes. Sharing in this way would be a tactical decision based on your intuition as to what might prove helpful to this particular client and not a "blurt" that you delivered without thought.

You might sometimes decide to share but you are not obliged to share. Nor should you feel that you are maintaining too great a distance or too stiff a demeanor by not sharing. You can be appropriately warm and close without ever revealing anything about yourself. Nor does your client really want to hear about you, since he believes that his experiences make him a unique case. You can lose a little of his trust and a little of his respect by telling stories about the time that this or that happened to you. So, share in a measured way, if you like, but also feel free not to share—that freedom not to have to share is another place of ease.

10. THE EASE OF LEAVING

In a practiced way, you leave your clients "at the office" rather than carrying them home with you. You don't dismiss them; you don't reject them; you don't sigh a deep sigh of relief as if some burden had been lifted off your shoulders. Rather, you quietly resume your life with its other meaning investments, meaning opportunities, life purpose choices, relaxations, errands, responsibilities, and all the rest.

You have a life that requires you. It may be the case that you can't leave family members and friends without provoking guilt in you but you can and must leave clients and not carry them about with you. This practiced leaving makes coming back to them that much easier. If you are keeping notes and records, do that quickly and on the spot; if you have other client-related chores that you must attend to, attend to them as quickly and easily as you can; and then be free and feel free when you shut the office door behind you.

This is good for your own mental health, good for the other people in your life, and something that you can legitimately do in a way that a lawyer up against a summation or an accountant up against an audit can't. In this sense, that you can have a real closing time and leave your work at the office, you have it easier than many other professionals who find themselves working around the clock nowadays.

These, then, are ten areas of ease. Of course, they don't make humane helping easy. But few jobs, careers, or callings are genuinely easy. There is nothing particularly easy about being an overworked physician, an underemployed actor, an under-inspired attorney, a bored office worker, a physically exhausted laborer, or a beleaguered teacher. And doing the same job—any job—for a few decades may well grow tiresome. In this context, that most work is work and that it becomes more like work over the long haul, humane helping may not prove harder than other work.

The setting in which we do our work may make it that much harder to provide humane help. A helper in a private practice setting who does not require or accept insurance payments is in a very different, presumably better position than, say, a psychiatric nurse on a locked ward or a psycho-therapist limited by insurance considerations, HMO rules, or (in the case of British helpers) the dictates of the National Health Service (NHS).

Likewise, the dominant paradigms of "doctors of the brain" and "doctors of the mind" make humane helping considerably harder. These two paradigms create "standards of care" with which you may disagree, proscribe you from engaging in interactions that you believe might prove useful, and hold the specter of legal sanctions over your head. But given that most work is hard and given that the ten places of ease I've described in this chapter are genuine saving graces, humane helping may strike you as well worth the effort involved.

POINTS FOR REFLECTION

1. What if your client wants to be "treated" or "cured" and you see your job as "helping"? How will you reconcile this difference in goals and objectives?

2. If one of your jobs is planting seeds, how will you know if those seeds ever flowered? Do you need to know?

3. Do you believe that a "small thing" that you say in session might actually help a lot? If so, what does that imply about the nature of your work?

4. Describe in your own language what "not striving" and "not attaching" in the context of helping means.

5. Are you impressed by these places of ease, does helping still seem quite hard, or a little of both?

NOTE

1 In personal correspondence dated April 2, 2017.

3 Embracing Not Knowing

You may know a lot by virtue of your experiences as a helper. You may have a very good idea of what helps a stubborn girl who isn't eating, anxious clients with a fear of flying, or clients in early recovery from an addiction. You may have a practiced way of sitting calmly, leaning forward, and listening that helps clients share what's troubling them. You may know a lot about the rhythms of working with human beings, a lot about using a particular method, or a lot about understanding a certain issue. Nevertheless, when it comes to helping with human issues like despair, anxiety, meaninglessness, and so on, we can never know another human being well enough to do what in medicine is done every single day.

In medicine, you cast a broken arm in a certain way because you can actually see the fracture and because you know that breaks knit in a particular way if you cast the arm appropriately. This is the essence of knowing and this is done every day in medicine. No equivalent knowing exists when it comes to human affairs, no matter how practiced, knowing, and wise you are as a helper. We don't know and can't know if and when a small thing in a person's life—the equivalent of a fly buzzing—might produce a huge effect. We don't know and can't know when and if a sudden insight might transform a person's outlook on life. We don't know and can't know what a person's sadness is really all about, even if we have some obvious candidates, like a lost love or a recent firing. Nor, despite our past successes, do we know what helping tactics to try that guarantee success with the person sitting across from us.

Picture the people you know very well, say your mother, father, brother, or sister. If you wanted your mother to experience less sadness, if you wanted your father to show more compassion, if you wanted your brother to take better charge of his life, if you wanted your sister to harm herself less, would you know what helping tactics to try that might come with anything like a guarantee of success—even if you've been a helping professional for a very long time? The answer is a resounding no. Certainly there are suggestions you might make and strategies you might try—but with anything like a guarantee of success? No, definitely and unfortunately not.

Given all that we don't know and can't know about the person sitting across from us, do we therefore say to him or her, "I have no idea"? In a careful and particular way, we do. We tell the truth, not for the sake of telling the truth but because it is both humane and helpful to do so. It matches what the person already knows, that no one, himself included, has anything like an accurate picture of his plight or of the causes of his plight. You can fool him with your brilliance or your practiced technique into believing that you know more than you do know—indeed, you can just put on a white coat and he is likely to believe what you have to say—but it is more humane and more helpful to tell the truth.

Why is that more humane? Because being fed humbug is alienating and adds to one's existential malaise and one's sense that life is a fraud. I remember when, as a young lad just out of the Army and working for the Veterans Administration as a benefits counselor, I was told by my supervisor to always say to a veteran filing for benefits, "You'll hear in about six to eight weeks." We were told to say that even if we knew that the veteran wouldn't hear about his benefits for six months or longer. Too much of life is like that and it sours us on institutions, on people, and on life itself. It would have been ever so much better to say, "I don't really know when you're going to hear—it may well take up to six months, if not longer." The first way makes no waves, ruffles no feathers, and is institutionally safe. The second way, though more jarring, is ultimately less alienating and more helpful.

Of course, you don't just come out and say to clients, "I have no idea!" You do not make a face and throw up your hands. Rather, you tie together one profound truth, about all that mutual not knowing, with a second profound truth, that there is still help available even though neither of you knows for sure or knows enough. You say things like "Let's see if we can figure this out" and "Where do you think we ought to focus?" and "What's your intuition about what might help?" You say, "Many folks do get less sad when they get a better grip on their thoughts" and "The following technique does seem to help a lot of people stop smoking" and all sorts of similar measured offers. In countless ways, you share these two truths, that neither of you can know for sure but that there are nevertheless things to try that might be of help.

And what if, when you say, "Where do you think we ought to focus?" your client throws up his hands and exclaims, "I have no idea!", followed by "You're the expert!"? In that case, you remind him of the basics. You say, "I know precious little about what's going inside of you, what you've been through, or what might work. You're going to have to help me a lot." You say, "I have some ideas about what might be going on and what might help and I'm willing to share my thoughts with you but that is not at all the same as me being an expert." You do not take the ball back that he has flung at you; you do not agree that you are the expert; and you remind him that you are not a plumber who fixes pipes but a person in conversation with another person.

Let's say that you're a psychotherapist and your client is a woman of forty-five who is complaining of fatigue, a variety of physical problems, and general unhappiness. Her adult children are experiencing their own problems, her husband is himself "depressed," and she has returned to the workforce after having been a stay-at-home mom. Her own parents, now that they have turned eighty, are experiencing new health problems and her mother recently fell, fracturing a shoulder and putting new burdens on your client, including the burden of dealing with her siblings who are not very interested in helping with their injured mother. Additionally, she is experiencing financial problems, existential malaise, and sadness over the state of the world.

This might be virtually any first-world middle-aged woman today. On the one hand, we have an immediate sense of what's wrong: all of the things she's named and more, no doubt. We would expect that she and her husband rarely have sexual relations; we would expect that she had some dream in childhood, maybe to be a dancer or a writer, that got deferred or that never panned out and that is still alive and aching; the list of additional sore points might prove very long. But even if we managed to create that complete list, and even if that list in some sense amounted to a decent summary of her current situation, would we really know if we'd missed something crucial or if, in choosing one thing on that list to work on, we'd picked the right sore point?

We couldn't possibly know. So, we patiently hang out in not knowing rather than rushing to simplify matters with a so-called diagnosis. In most settings, this client would certainly—and virtually instantly—end up with a depression diagnosis, which would likely be followed by a regimen of so-called antidepressants. In one gulp an abrupt movement would have been made from genuine not knowing to "knowing clearly" that this woman's primary challenge was something called a "clinical depression." Since this abrupt movement reflects the current paradigm and the current standard of care, practitioners are pressured to proceed in exactly this way. Sitting with this woman, you might be quite well aware that you don't know enough yet—and yet suddenly there you are "diagnosing and treating a clinical depression."

Let's say that you could make yourself hang out in not knowing and, instead of "diagnosing," just chat. What might you learn? You and she might discover that her return to the workforce is making her extremely anxious, much more anxious than she realized. You and she might discover that her concerns about her adult children are more pressing than she realized and are actually on her mind day and night. You and she might discover that she's been dealing with a lifetime of sadness and discontent connected to her unhappy childhood. You and she might discover that her thwarted desire to pursue a certain dream or to live a certain life still weighs heavily on her and is in some sense coming to a head. Neither of you would have known any of this clearly until you in fact did know, until that particular insight crystallized through conversation and investigation. If you do not spend the necessary time, you and she might never know.

A diagnosis tends to foreclose on useful investigations of this sort. But even if you do manage to avoid diagnosing and even if you do hang out in not knowing, you may still remain quite in the dark after you converse and after you investigate. You may both still not know. The roots of her difficulties may remain unnamed and the difficulties themselves may be hard to pin down. What if her deep fatigue is connected to all those novels that never got written, what if that connection remains obscured, and what if that fatigue gets ascribed to an unhealthy diet or to poor sleep habits? In such a way might the two of you end up on the path of focusing a lot on diet or sleep habits and not on those unwritten novels. In this common, inadvertent, and unfortunate way you might miss the main challenge, because when dealing with real human beings much opaqueness often remains.

You must be easy with this truth, that even after wide-ranging and heartfelt investigations you may still not know enough and may end up focusing on some aspect of your client's life that isn't her main or deepest challenge. This will happen. In addition to a common outcome of that sort, it may also be the case that the person sitting across from you may not be making much of an effort to help herself. This frequent reality, usually conceptualized as resistance or defensiveness, makes helping that much more difficult. When you couple all that not knowing with your client not helping, that is quite a predicament. Yet you can still remain humane and helpful.

ONE PLACE OF NOT KNOWING: MANIA

Was there something in your training that helped you understand what "mania" is? I sincerely doubt it. Yet you are supposed to "diagnose bipolar disorder" by virtue of the presence of certain "symptoms"—without having the least clue what "mania" actually is. What an odd—and illegitimate—enterprise.

What is mania? The following is one unconventional view for your consideration. I take "mania" to be a state where a person's racing brain, already racing, races even faster, races out of control, and can sometimes race right off the tracks. Mania in my view is not a medical illness but a state of pressure and a state of siege.

A person's brain begins to race because it has been set in motion for all sorts of everyday reasons and as a result of multiple pressures. Then something additional occurs, very often an existential crisis, resulting in a dangerous increase in speed. It is this added pressure on top of already-existing pressure that causes the thing called mania.

I've worked with creative and performing artists as a therapist and as a creativity coach for more than thirty years and their concerns interest me a lot. One of those concerns is the thing commonly called "mania." People who are creative and who think a lot are more prone to so-called mania than people who do not think a lot and who aren't creative. This fact, which is indeed a fact, should alert us to the possibility that mania is not some pseudo-medical condition or some brain abnormality but a function of the real mental pressures put on individuals who use their brains and who rely on their brains.

That intelligent, creative, and thoughtful people are the ones more regularly afflicted by the thing called mania is beyond question. Research shows, for example, a clear linkage between achieving top grades and "bipolar disorder" (that is, that "disorder" where "depression" and "mania" cyclically appear), between scoring high on tests and "bipolar disorder," and between similar measures of mental accomplishment, brainpower, and mania.

There is a great deal of evidence supporting the idea that mania disproportionately affects smart, creative, thoughtful people. One study involving 700,000 adults and reported in the *British Journal of Psychiatry* indicated that former straight-A students were four times more likely to be "bipolar" (or "manic-depressive") than those who had achieved lower grades. Are these folks "more ill" than their C-average counterparts or are they putting their brains under relatively more pressure, thereby causing dangerous speeding accidents? Which seems more likely to you? (*The Telegraph*, 2010)

In another study, individuals who scored the highest on tests for "mathematical reasoning" were at a twelve-times greater risk for "contracting bipolar disorder."[1] Similar studies underline the linkage between creativity and mania and we have thousands of years of anecdotal evidence to support the contention that smart and creative people often get manic (think of Virginia Woolf). Doesn't all this evidence suggest that enlisting your brain—say, to write a novel or to solve a riddle in theoretical physics—is a rather dangerous act, since it increases the pressure on a brain already pressured to deal with everyday matters like financial difficulties, psychological threats, and just finding your car keys?

Mania in my view is a racing brain driven extra fast—and ultimately too fast—by added pressures, needs, or impulses. Your brain was already racing; now it is racing dangerously. Because of these added pressures, anything that gets in the way of this felt forward motion—a physical obstacle, another person's viewpoint, even a delay in the bus arriving—is viewed as a tremendous irritation. Hence the irritability so often associated with mania. This irritation makes perfect sense: if you *must* get on with whatever your dangerously racing brain is proposing—to get every wall painted red, to capture that song you're trying to compose, to solve that theorem you've been working on for six months—*then nothing must get in the way.*

It is this "must" that is at the heart of mania and that turns an everyday racing brain into one that begins to race out of control. This "must" is the heavy foot on the pedal that is driving that racing brain too fast. There is a sense of emergency here, most often an existential emergency as the individual stares at nothingness and is petrified by the view. She must get away from that horrible feeling and with a strangled laugh that mimics mirth but that isn't mirth she turns to her brain for help; and in order to help her, protect her, and even save her, it goes into overdrive.

She is frightened by that whiff of the void and, in anguish and in order to deal with all that existential danger, she shouts to her brain, "Get me out of here!" Her brain takes off, dreaming up every manner of scheme, activity, and desire. But you really can't keep accelerating your brain, even if you're doing so in order to stave off meaninglessness, because your brain can (and sometimes does) derail. You must deal with existential danger in a different way; if you don't, you'll experience "symptoms of mania" and, among other unfortunate results, acquire a mental disorder label.

All of the characteristic "symptoms of mania" that we see, including (apparently) high spirits, heightened sexual appetite, high arousal levels, high energy levels, sweating, pacing, sleeplessness, and, at its severest, when the train has run off the rails, hallucinations, delusions of grandeur, suspiciousness, aggression, and wild, self-defeating plans and schemes, make perfect sense when viewed from the perspective that a powerful pressure, likely existential in nature, has supercharged a brain already feverishly racing along. Your powerful thinking machine rushes off to handle this emergency and all the "symptoms of mania" naturally follow.

This contention, that added pressure, often existential in nature, is causing an already racing brain to race all that much faster, much better fits the observable facts than do any "mental disorder" or "broken machinery" hypotheses. What we are observing is a human being *under tremendous pressure*, someone who is attempting to relieve that tremendous pressure by talking a mile a minute, by having lots of sex, by dreaming up grandiose schemes, by running around naked, or by engaging in some other "manic" activity. That brain isn't broken; rather, it is on a wild, ineffective mission to save its owner.

What, then, might help? First, anything that reduces the speed at which your brain races; and second, entering into a different relationship with meaning so that fewer existential crises occur. As to the first, we know lots of things to try, for example mindfulness techniques that help you learn how to quiet your mind. Studies show exactly that, that negative consequences of a racing brain such as insomnia are reduced through mindfulness training. For example, studies run by Cynthia Gross and her colleagues at the University of Minnesota showed that after eight weeks of mindfulness training participants fell asleep more quickly than a group taking "sleep medication"—and had the benefits last over time (Gross et al., 2011).

Mindfulness techniques are extremely valuable. Equally important is threat reduction. Threats cause your brain to race; when you reduce or, better still, when you eliminate the threats that you're facing, your brain can be less vigilant and can relax. You can meditate for an hour every morning but if, when your husband comes home he insults you and criticizes you, your meditation practice probably won't prove enough. A divorce may be needed. If you experience your profession as meaningless, your meditation practice will probably prove insufficient. In order to calm your racing brain, you may need to change your life so that you feel less threatened, less sad, less anxious, less upset with life, less self-reproachful, and so on. All of these changes for the better amount to a braking mechanism for a racing brain.

There are many things to try to reduce the pressure on your brain and thereby have it speed less. One crucial effort is making sure that you understand how meaning operates, the extent to which you can both coax it into existence and live for periods without it, and why living your life purpose choices is the best guarantee that you'll experience life as meaningful. Getting all-around smart about existential matters is crucial: understanding how you can make the shift from seeking meaning to making meaning, how you can live day-in and day-out as a value-based meaning-maker, and how you can avoid meaning crises and deal with them when they occur.

Is this anything like a correct view of mania? I have no idea. Do you? We do not actually know and we aren't close to knowing. Therefore, it is reasonable that we might feel frustrated and daunted when dealing with a person in such a state. But we should also take some pride in the fact that we are not fooling ourselves into believing that observing some "symptoms of mania" is anything like understanding mania.

Say that your client claims to "know" what is troubling her but what she presents as an explanation strikes you as coy, incomplete, unconvincing, or mistaken. If the woman I described above were to collapse all of the challenges she reported into the claim that it's "all about my hormones" or that it's "just that I can't get a good night's sleep," you would be right to presume that this is too limited a labeling and explanation of her difficulties.

Naturally you wouldn't flat-out dispute her contention. But you might well say, "No doubt that's a part of it. But there must be an awful lot we don't know yet about what's going on, don't you think?" You would underline the fact that neither of you know enough yet; you would carefully dispute her oversimplification; and by so doing you would create an opening for a deeper conversation that sometimes will indeed follow.

And what if you can't reach the person sitting across from you? What if your mutual not knowing is coupled with your client's staunch lack of helpfulness? What if he demands to be fixed, maintains a steadfast disinterest in his own well-being, is very attached to his addictions, obsessions, and habits, is looking for answers of the sort that a diagnosis seem to afford, or is in some other way difficult, defensive, disengaged, or unavailable? What then?

This is another aspect of the reality of not knowing: of not knowing what to do with an unhelpful client. The most usual results of this particular dynamic are coercion or quick fixes. As a humane helper, however, you do not have to opt for coercion or a quick fix, nor do you have to throw up your hands in dismay or consternation. Rather, you continue to try to be of help—maybe in a very direct sort of way, given his unhelpfulness. To a court-mandated, driving under the influence (DUI) counseling group participant, you might say, "I don't hear you taking any responsibility for drinking excessively. Which means your problems are likely to

continue, don't you think?" With a despairing, shut-down, uncommu-
nicative client, you might say, "I see how terribly sad you are. Is there
anything at all you can tell me about what's going on?" You are hoping
that such "interventions" will help while fully recognizing that the person
across from you may not respond.

You surrender to the reality that knowing another person is very
different from knowing the solution to a math puzzle and you likewise
surrender to the reality that your client may be thoroughly invested in
preventing you from knowing what he's thinking or feeling. In life, we
like to know; it can bother us tremendously not to know and can even
cause us acute anxiety. As a helping professional, however, you have
chosen a "not knowing" profession. You might have gone into accounting
or math teaching but you didn't. All your classes, internships, degrees,
licenses, and life experiences notwithstanding, you picked a profession
where not knowing is the norm. All of that not knowing that you are
bound to face may test your patience and your nerves but surrendering
to that truth may also increase your compassion. Not knowing certainly
muddles matters but it need not defeat you.

FOUR REMINDERS ABOUT NOT KNOWING

1. In working as a helping professional, you will know less than you
    wish you knew. This is an inevitable feature of working with human
    beings.

2. There is a strong temptation to reduce the anxiety of not knowing
    by acting as if you do know, for instance by acting like an expert and
    proclaiming a diagnosis. A humane helper watches out for this
    natural tendency and hangs out in not knowing rather than opting
    for too-easy, formulaic knowing.

3. Despite all that you do not know, you can still be of help.

4. Your client may prove uncooperative and unhelpful. This further
    reduces your ability to be of help but it does not render helping
    impossible. Even if you do not know enough and even if your client
    is being his or her tricky, difficult human self, by employing your
    practiced helping tactics and by remaining present and engaged, you
    may well still prove of help.

POINTS FOR REFLECTION

1. Explain in your own language why the humane way is admitting that we don't know what we don't know.

2. How easy or hard do you expect it will be to hang out in not knowing? What might make it easier?

3. Pick something about which you know very little, for example "mania." How might you learn more? And what do you suspect might be the limits of your knowing?

4. What might you try when neither you nor your client knows what exactly is troubling her?

5. How will you deal with the reality that you are bound to know less than you wish you knew?

NOTE

1 Wrong Planet Community Chat Forum, December 16, 2013.

REFERENCES

Gross, C. R., Kreitzer, M. J., Reilly-Spong, M., Wall, M., Winbush, N. Y., Patterson, R., . . . Cramer-Bornemann, M. (2011). Mindfulness-Based Stress Reduction Versus Pharmacotherapy for Chronic Primary Insomnia: A Randomized Controlled Clinical Trial. *EXPLORE: The Journal of Science and Healing*, 7(2), 76–87. doi:10.1016/j.explore.2010.12.003

Straight-A schoolchildren at higher risk of bipolar disorder, research claims. (2010, Jan. & Feb.). *The Telegraph*. Retrieved May & June, 2017, from www.telegraph. co.uk/news/health/news/7137591/Straight-A-schoolchildren-at-higher-risk-of-bipolar-disorder-research-claims.html

4 On Not Diagnosing

An important step in the direction of humane helping is sidestepping the pseudo-scientific, pseudo-medical enterprise of "diagnosing and treating mental disorders" and instead helping people meet their challenges without unnecessarily labeling them and without sending them in the direction of controversial chemical fixes. This is not to say that there can never be a place for so-called psychiatric medication—we'll chat more about this issue separately—but a humane helper might well decide that as a general rule she will disavow chemical fixes.

A humane helper, as I'm describing her, takes a critical stance with respect to the current dominant paradigm that analogizes from medicine and, without scientific or logical justification and hand-in-hand with pharmaceutical companies, brazenly creates disingenuous categories of mental disorders meant to mimic the genuine categories of physical disorders. If she is one sort of helper, say if she is a life coach, she can do this sidestepping relatively easily. If she is another sort of helper, for instance if she is a psychiatrist or clinical psychologist, she will find this movement away from illegitimate labeling and wanton chemical dispensing much harder to accomplish. Whatever her designation, she ought to inform herself about what critics of the current dominant paradigm, as embodied in the DSM and the International Classification of Diseases (ICD), are saying.

What are they saying? Gary Greenberg practices psychotherapy in Connecticut, is a contributing editor for *Harper's Magazine*, and is the author of four books, including *Manufacturing Depression: The Secret History of a Modern Disease* and *The Book of Woe: The*

DSM and the Unmaking of Psychiatry. Gary explained to me in an interview:

> The DSM, the Diagnostic and Statistical Manual of Mental Disorders, is the American Psychiatric Association's compendium of psychiatric diagnoses. It lays out, dictionary-like, all the mental illnesses recognized by the APA [American Psychiatric Association], and the criteria by which they are known. Designed to provide a universal language for psychiatry, it is used by clinicians and researchers around the world.
>
> As a result of its predominance, the DSM's categories and concepts frame the discussion, within the mental health professions and in the general public, of mental suffering. When a person in casual conversation describes herself as "totally OCD [obsessive compulsive disorder]" or when a teacher suggests to parents that they have their child evaluated for ADHD, they are, generally without knowing it, drawing on the DSM's categories.
>
> The DSM is very good at what it explicitly sets out to be good at, which is systematically describing the ways people suffer. A clinician tells another clinician that a patient has paranoid schizophrenia; assuming the diagnosis is made carefully, and assuming the second clinician is familiar with the diagnosis, then it is likely that useful information has been transmitted. Similarly, if a researcher publishes a paper about bipolar disorder, then it is safe to assume that he or she is writing about the same collection of symptoms that are the subject of other papers on bipolar disorder.
>
> The DSM, in other words, has scientific reliability (although not as much as is generally thought, and less in the DSM-5 than in previous recent editions). But it does not have scientific validity. The categories in it are constructs; there is no evidence that, for example, major depressive disorder exists in the same way that, say, diabetes or cancer exist. The disorders are purely heuristic. This aspect of the DSM, which is acknowledged by the APA, becomes a flaw when the diagnoses are reified and people, clinicians and the public alike, begin to think of them as real. At that point, what is, at best, an anthropology of mental suffering becomes a pseudoscience.
>
> This outcome is not accidental, or the result of ignorance. Since the third edition came out in 1980, its implicit purpose has been to provide scientific respectability to psychiatry, which has long suffered from

"physics envy." The DSM-III adopted a scientific rhetoric, but without providing an actual scientific basis for its rendering of the world of mental illness. This move succeeded in restoring the credibility of psychiatry, but the authority it derives as a result is not really backed up by the kind of science that backs up, say, cancer research. Psychiatry's reach, as embodied in the DSM, exceeds its grasp.

(Maisel, 2016a)

Peter R. Breggin, MD, has been called "the conscience of psychiatry" for his many decades of successful efforts to reform the mental health field. He has authored dozens of scientific articles and more than twenty books including *Talking Back to Prozac* (with Ginger Breggin); *Medication Madness: The Role of Psychiatric Drugs in Cases of Violence, Suicide and Crime*; *Psychiatric Drug Withdrawal: A Guide for Prescribers, Therapists, Patients and Their Families*; and *Guilt, Shame and Anxiety: Understanding and Overcoming Negative Emotions*. Peter explained to me in an interview:

I began attacking the medical model, including diagnoses and physical treatments, decades ago. Many people continue to benefit from one of my earlier books about it, called *Toxic Psychiatry: Why Therapy, Empathy and Love Must Replace the Drugs, Electroshock, and Biochemical Theories of the "New Psychiatry."* The psychiatric model of human suffering has caused untold damage to hundreds of millions of victims of involuntary treatment, psychiatric hospitals, drugs, and electroshock.

It has also set back civilization by undermining Western traditions of individuality, personal responsibility, and love. It has convinced modern society that emotional suffering is based in so-called biochemical imbalances when in reality it is rooted in a complex combination of human nature, individual experience and choice-making, and societal influences. This flawed biological model ignores all the important realities in human life from the dreadful effects of childhood trauma and adult disappointment and loss to the importance of living by worthwhile principles and ideals.

(Maisel, 2016c)

Joanna Moncrieff is a Senior Lecturer at University College London and also works as a consultant psychiatrist in the NHS in London. Her academic work consists of a critical appraisal of drug treatment for mental health problems, as well as work on the history, philosophy, and politics of psychiatry and mental health. She makes a clear distinction between a disease-centered model of drug action, where actual diseases exist and are being treated, and a drug-centered model of drug action, where chemicals with powerful effects are employed to produce certain effects (as often negative as positive). She argues that the former is what the current paradigm purports to be engaged in and that the latter is what is actually going on. She explained to me in an interview:

> The idea of diagnosis [in the mental health field] is misleading. The DSM and ICD are classification systems, not diagnostic systems. They are attempts to organize the myriad of mental health "symptoms" or problems into categories, based on our experience of the sort of patterns that people manifest.
>
> Classifications do not indicate the causes of conditions, they are merely a way of organizing experience, and they are highly subjective. Mental health problems are highly individual, so there is no universally valid or useful way of classifying them. Pre-determined categories do not capture the essence of a particular individual's problems, and rarely tell you much that is useful.
>
> The problem with our current approach to treatment is that it is presented as targeting a putative underlying brain disease or abnormality. It is based on a presumption that drugs act according to the disease-centered model of drug action. Therefore, we have ignored the psychoactive (mind-altering) properties of the drugs we use. We should have a greater knowledge of all the alterations that drugs produce in body and mind. The psychoactive properties of some drugs may be useful in some situations, but they can also be unpleasant and disabling, and this is not recognized widely enough.
>
> (Maisel, 2016b)

CHEMICALS AND THEIR PLACE

A humane helper who is operating in today's environment needs to know what she thinks about the use of so-called psychiatric medication to treat so-called mental disorders, diseases, and illnesses. Because so many millions of people have received a diagnosis and a subsequent prescription, because these numbers are only increasing (especially among children), and because virtually every client she sees will be on one or more of these so-called meds or may be anticipating having a conversation about them, she is obliged to understand what is going on and to stake out her position.

It won't really do for her to shake her head and say, "I stay away from all that" or to try to diplomatically straddle the fence with the pronouncement, "No doubt medication has its place." She must know more than that and, quite likely, say more than that. This is an area where a humane helper ought to educate herself, starting, I would suggest, with books like Joanna Moncrieff's *The Myth of the Chemical Cure*, Robert Whitaker's *Anatomy of an Epidemic*, and my *The Future of Mental Health*.

Medicine is wonderful. But the chemicals employed to "treat mental disorders" are not medicine. Not every chemical used by a person to create an effect can rightly be called medicine. If we use language this loosely and call every chemical with a powerful effect a medication then we have completely bastardized language and made a mockery of the ideas of disease and of medication. Biologically altering our experience of life via chemicals is not the same as treating illnesses with drugs.

Human beings have used chemicals to alter their experience of life since the beginning of time. Peyote, magic mushrooms, Scotch, marijuana, cocaine, nicotine, caffeine, heroin, wine: the list of chemicals used by human beings for the purpose of feeling different is very long. It is only metaphoric—and a profoundly dangerous and ill-chosen metaphor—to call these "medications that treat the disease of life." You can call these chemicals sacred, dangerous, a blessing, a problem, or whatever else you like: just don't call them medicine.

Would you accept that the word "medicine" has been appropriately used in any of the following contexts? From a killer: "Arsenic is the medicine I use to treat the disease of being alive from which my victims regularly suffer." From a safari guide: "Tranquilizer darts are the medicine I use to treat the animals I encounter who are suffering from the disease of wanting to eat me."

From a bar patron: "Scotch is the medicine I use to treat my disease of having a wife I can't stand."

If a mental health provider makes no effort to identify the cause of your suffering—if he is completely indifferent as to whether you are suffering from a life problem, a feature of your formed or your original personality, a reaction to your circumstances, a psychological issue, or a biological issue—if he makes zero effort and simply says "we call your symptom picture a mental disorder and we medicate it," you should treat his utterance with disdain and not accept the word "medicate" in that sentence.

That isn't to say that you may not want what a chemical dispenser is offering. The safari guide may get great, life-saving value from his tranquilizer darts. You may want a certain effect even if you have no mental disorder. You may want a tranquilizer to deal with anxiety even if you don't have "the mental disorder of generalized anxiety." Of course, you might also decide that you don't want that tranquilizer. You may want a mood-altering substance to deal with your chronic sadness even if you don't have "the mental disorder of clinical depression." Of course, you might also decide that you don't want that mood-altering substance. If a chemical is available that has a certain powerful effect and you desire that effect, if you also believe that it really has that effect (it may only have a placebo effect), and if you likewise also believe that its positive value outweighs its risks, then that chemical is yours for the taking. Just think twice (or three times)—and don't call it medicine.

What is our humane helper to do with this really difficult conundrum: that she may understand clearly that "psychiatric medication" isn't medicine while also understanding that many human beings might want the powerful effects that these chemicals afford? What sort of line ought she to walk as she works with the suffering human being sitting across from her? And if she tries to explain all this to him, might that even put her at some legal or professional risk, given that the current "standard of care" is based on the idea of "diagnosing mental disorders and, once diagnosed, treating them with drugs"?

There are three camps in the mental health field with respect to so-called psychiatric medications. There are those who prescribe them and who advocate for them, whether or not they one hundred percent believe in them (these are primarily but not exclusively psychiatrists). There are those who believe that so-called psychiatric medications are something rather different from medicine—namely chemicals with powerful effects—who see some place for those powerful effects, if only their rationale were differently and honestly presented, and who discuss these matters with their clients. And then there are those, the vast majority, who stay mute on the subject and dodge the subject and by doing so tacitly and functionally support the current chemical-dispensing paradigm.

What if, as a humane helper, you find yourself in the second camp and want to share your opinions with the human being sitting across from you? What is the right, smart, best, or safest thing to do in that situation, given that the person you are working with might possibly benefit from the chemical in question, its downside notwithstanding? While we wait for a different future, one where our lack of knowledge is generally admitted, where opinions of this sort are safe to share, and where some new, extensive research project has been launched that moves our understanding forward, what can a humane helper in this position do right now?

It would be excellent if humane helpers were permitted to say their piece. It should not have to prove legally dangerous or professionally dangerous to call these chemicals with powerful effects what they indubitably are, mere chemicals with powerful effects and not actual drugs. But currently all of the power and leverage are on the side of the mental health establishment. Each humane helper will need to find her own way and her own talking points in this treacherous area, while, one hopes, supporting her fellow professionals who speak out and advocate for change.

Compounding this problem is the following. Can a person who is severely sad, intensely anxious, actively "manic," or "psychotic," or who for some reason is invested in believing that he has a mental disorder that requires medication, really be expected to listen to a humane helper's complicated explanations and distinctions or to know what to do if handed a choice this confusing? Could even a highly educated, relatively undisturbed person make sense of this choice or know how to proceed? Wouldn't you, yourself, feel at sea trying to decide if a given chemical really was or wasn't medication and really was or wasn't likely to help you?

In a better future that I can envision but don't expect to see, these chemicals, and more like them that are no doubt coming, might still be available and might prove helpful to some people. They just wouldn't be called medicine; their logic would become exposed and transparent; and new, better conversations about their use or their avoidance would prove possible. In that better future, a humane helper would have a much easier time of staking out her position with respect to these chemicals. Right now, she will not find it easy making her way among the boulders.

Here are additional voices that a humane helper ought to hear. Peter Kinderman is a professor of Clinical Psychology at the University of Liverpool, current President of the British Psychological Society, and the author of *A Prescription for Psychiatry*. Peter explained to me in an interview:

I believe that mental health services should be based on the premise that the origins of distress are largely social. The guiding idea underpinning mental health services needs to change from an assumption that our role is to treat "disease" to an appreciation that our role is to help and support people who are distressed as a result of their life circumstances, and how they have made sense of and reacted to them. This also means that we should replace "diagnoses" with straightforward descriptions of problems. We must stop regarding people's very real emotional distress as merely the symptom of diagnosable "illnesses."

This does not mean rejecting rigor or the scientific method—quite the reverse. We can straightforwardly define people's problems—it's what scientists do—and this would have greater scientific validity and would be more than sufficient as a basis for individual care planning and for the design and planning of services. Our health services should sharply reduce our reliance on medication to address emotional distress. We should not look to medication to "cure" or even "manage" non-existent underlying "illnesses." We must offer services that help people to help themselves and each other rather than disempowering them.

That means involving a wide range of community workers and psychologists in multidisciplinary teams, and promoting psychosocial rather than medical solutions. Where individual therapy is needed, effective, formulation-based, and therefore individually tailored, psychological therapies should be available to all. When people are in acute crisis, residential care may be needed, but this should not be seen as a medical issue. Adopting this approach would result in a fundamental shift from a medical to a psychosocial focus. And because experiences of neglect, rejection, and abuse are hugely important in the genesis of many problems, we need to redouble our efforts to address the underlying issues of abuse, discrimination and social inequity.

(Maisel, 2016d)

The document that serves as the labeling bible for American mental health professionals and for many other professionals as well is the DSM. Much of the rest of the world relies on a different document, the ICD. Both documents as they relate to so-called mental disorders are flawed at best and fraudulent at worst. The definition of a mental disorder presented in these documents is purposefully vacuous and all embracing; the logic of diagnosing a mental disorder based on symptom pictures, rather than on causes, is illegitimate; and the fact that not a word is breathed about either the causes of the disorders described or about how to treat the disorders described further invalidates them.

In these documents and in the model and paradigm they support, human experiences of a certain sort have been transformed for money into pseudo-medical mental disorder labels. For example, when you're in despair you receive a "depression" label and then a chemical called an "anti-depressant." That someone has labeled another person depressed or bipolar or disordered in some way only means that they have affixed a label to that person, not that they have genuinely diagnosed some actually existing medical condition. As a humane helper, it is squarely on your shoulders to understand these controversies and criticisms and come to your own informed conclusions.

Consider the following strong sentiment. The French psychiatrist and psychoanalyst Alain Vanier, a professor at the University of Paris, explained to me:[1]

Psychiatric systems of classification have no scientific basis. Psychiatry has never been able to fully rely on the anatomical-clinical method the way other medical specialties have done. Modern psychiatry is under the illusion that such verification can be obtained through brain imaging, which would function as a kind of virtual anatomical-clinical method. But this research, which can in itself be of some interest, is far from giving us a tool that we could use to establish a classification.

In other words, all classifications [in psychiatry] are necessarily cultural and depend on the way in which the given society deals with "mental illness." No doubt the current proliferation of diagnoses, followed by an expanded use of medication, makes the pharmaceutical industry very happy, but it should lead us to ask ourselves the fundamental question, namely what is it that makes today's world so unbearable for so many people?

Clinicians possess tremendous power to diagnose based on what many consider a mere whim. Rachel Cooper, a senior lecturer in Philosophy at Lancaster University, UK and author of the book *Diagnosing the Diagnostic and Statistical Manual of Mental Disorders*, explained to me in an interview:

As an example of this whimsical power, consider the DSM-5 diagnostic criteria for phobia. In DSM-IV diagnosed individuals had to recognize their fears as unreasonable. In DSM-5 the fear merely has to be judged by the clinician to be out of proportion. I think the revision was a mistake. Consider what can now happen if someone develops rational fears on the basis of information that the diagnosing clinician lacks.

Take a scientist working on avian flu whose studies lead her to the conclusion that a worldwide pandemic is imminent. She comes to develop rational fears about sick birds. Using DSM-IV criteria she did not have a phobia, as she would not have considered her fears unreasonable. Using DSM-5, if a clinician (who we will suppose knows nothing of these matters) judges her fear as being out of proportion, she can receive a diagnosis. This seems wrong.

(Maisel, 2016e)

This power to diagnose the presence of a "mental disorder," "mental illness," or "mental disease" has been used coercively throughout history. Historically you were labeled with a mental disorder if you were a homosexual, if you were a slave and didn't like it, if you were a "hysterical" woman, if you were a Jew in Nazi Germany, if you were a dissident in the Soviet Union, if you were a "feebleminded Indian"—and now if you are a squirming third-grade boy bored out of your wits. It is no friendly, helpful gesture that a clinician is engaged in when he or she diagnoses you. To a very large extent, it is a sociopolitical statement.

Our humane helper will educate herself about these matters and get savvy. As she does, she will want to make the basic shift in her own mind from "mental disease thinking" to "problems in living thinking." Rather than automatically ticking off squirming as a "symptom" of the "mental disorder of ADHD" or gloominess as a "symptom" of the "mental disorder of clinical depression," she will train herself to ask the question, "I wonder why little Johnny is squirming?" or "I wonder why Jane is gloomy?" She will begin to lead with "What's going on?" rather than with "What mental disorder can I detect?" and stop looking for mental disorders just because shopping catalogs for mental disorders, the DSM and the ICD, happen to exist.

Richard Pemberton, former chair of the Division of Clinical Psychology of the British Psychological Society, and Tony Wainwright explain in the *International Journal of Clinical and Health Psychology*:

> While biology plays a mediating role in all human experiences, mental distress is not best understood as disease process, and this particular paradigm has comprehensively failed in the field of psychiatry ... Mental Health theory and practice is at a crossroads. The language and categories we use to describe psychological distress are changing and as evidenced by the furor over DSM-5 are being challenged from all sides. The complex interplay between the physical, the psychological, the social and cultural is always likely to be controversial and prone to change.
>
> We however have argued that it is time that the current disease-based systems are replaced. We advocate using the advances in our understanding of the psychological, social and physical mechanisms that underpin psychological wellbeing and mental distress to change the way we respond at a community and an individual level. ... [And] we need to be careful that we don't just replace disease-based frameworks with overly restrictive psychological ones. Success will include social inclusion in the local community, friendships within and outside of the mental health system, and purpose in life.
>
> (Pemberton and Wainwright, 2014)

Suffering isn't a medical condition. It would be pretty to think that there can be pills to treat life but that just isn't possible. Indeed, our everyday wishful thinking for easy remedies does a beautiful job of propping up the drug companies' campaigns that try to sell us on the notion that everything unwanted, from anxiety ruining your erection to your boss stealing away another one of your weekends, has a chemical answer. These challenges aren't medical conditions; suffering and distress aren't medical conditions. As a humane helper, try to get clear in your own mind what you think about the very idea of "diagnosing mental disorders." You may discover that the "no diagnosing whatsoever" option makes the most sense to you.

POINTS FOR REFLECTION

1. Given that the DSM and the ICD are the main props that support the current dominant paradigm that "mental disorders" exist and that they can be "diagnosed" via "symptom pictures," what are your thoughts on these two influential documents?

2. To what extent do you believe that there ought to be proof that a "mental disorder" exists before it is said to exist? What proof would you like to see that you would consider compelling?

3. Describe in your own language the distinction between "medication" and "chemicals with powerful effects." Do you have an opinion into which category "psychiatric medication" falls?

4 If it is part of your job to "diagnose and treat mental disorders" but you don't believe much in that model or paradigm, how will you walk that line?

5. Present your view on how you might help clients without engaging in any "diagnosing" at all.

NOTE

1 Alain Vanier in personal correspondence with Eric Maisel, dated May 21, 2016.

REFERENCES

Maisel, E. (2016a). "Gary Greenberg on Manufacturing Depression." *Psychology Today* www.psychologytoday.com/blog/rethinking-mental-health/201603/gary-greenberg-manufacturing-depression

Maisel, E. (2016b). "Joanna Moncrieff on the Myth of the Chemical Cure." *Psychology Today*. www.psychologytoday.com/blog/rethinking-mental-health/201602/joanna-moncrieff-the-myth-the-chemical-cure

Maisel, E. (2016c). "Peter Breggin on the Psycho-Pharmaceutical Complex." *Psychology Today*. www.psychologytoday.com/blog/rethinking-mental-health/201604peter-breggin-the-psycho-pharmaceutical-complex

Maisel, E. (2016d). "Peter Kinderman on the British Psychological Society." *Psychology Today*. www.psychologytoday.com/blog/rethinking-mental-health/201603/peter-kinderman-the-british-psychological-society

Maisel, E. (2016e). "Rachel Cooper on Classifying Madness and Diagnosing the DSM." *Psychology Today*. www.psychologytoday.com/blog/rethinking-mental-health/201604/rachel-cooper-classifying-madness-and-diagnosing-the-dsm

Maisel, E. (2016f). *The Future of Mental Health: Deconstructing the Mental Disorder Paradigm*. New Brunswick, NJ: Transaction Publishers.

Moncrieff, J. (2008). *The Myth of the Chemical Cure: A Critique of Psychiatric Drug Treatment*. Basingstoke: Palgrave Macmillan.

Pemberton, R. and Wainwright, T. (2014). "The End of Mental Illness Thinking?" *International Journal of Clinical and Health Psychology*, 14(3), 216–220.

Whitaker, R. (2010). *Anatomy of an Epidemic: Magic Bullets, Psychiatric Drugs, and the Astonishing Rise of Mental Illness in America*. New York: Crown Publishers.

5 Being with a Person

As a young therapist, I began working with a client named Sally. Sally made a point of saying nothing in session. Sally had a certain way of smiling that seemed to say, "I really do wish I had something to say, but I just don't." Sometimes we sat there for a whole session in silence. I had never experienced such silence before and I could hardly tolerate it. But I knew that I had something to learn from managing to sit there and "just be there" with Sally. And it wasn't easy!

Her silences were hard. Then, when she began speaking several sessions later, her speaking was hard. Suicidal thoughts, violent threats, sexual fantasies, horrible childhood abuse, and much more. What helper doesn't harbor the desire to refer Sally to "someone"? But who is that someone? We, the humane helpers, are the ones on the front lines of this distress and difficulty. And we have to be there, as calmly, patiently, and compassionately as we are able to be.

What is a therapist "supposed to do" when he or she first meets a client? According to textbooks on what should happen in the first session of psychotherapy, a diligent therapist should come away knowing his client's presenting problems, current mental status, mental health history and personal history, symptom pictures with respect to any syndromes that may be present (from depression and substance abuse to spiritual problems), red-flag issues like child abuse, elder abuse, suicidality, and dangerousness, and so much more that a therapist might be inclined to wonder, "When do I just relax, relate, and listen?"

The demands to gather information and to provide a diagnosis, demands exacerbated by managed care and brief therapy pressures, are only two of the many obstacles to the formation of a genuine human-feeling relationship between humane helper and client. A helper is likely to inadvertently put up walls, preach rather than interact, immediately problem-solve rather than listen, offer up theories rather than co-create understanding, dismiss her client's concerns and feelings, and engage in other efforts to remain safe and in charge. Between the demands to gather information and to provide a diagnosis and the many shadows in a helper's personality, simple relating often gets lost.

Rather than engage in efforts to avoid genuine human interactions, a humane helper will want to "join" with her clients. "Joining" is a practiced combination of being present, feeling empathetic, being interested in the other person, having some kindly feelings toward the other person, and hoping and intending to be of help—while at the same time studiously maintaining excellent boundaries and carefully not getting over-invested in her client's dramas.

Say that you're a creativity coach, one sort of helper with whom I'm very familiar. Can you feel the hold the drug habit has on the rock musician sitting across from you? Can you feel what it's like for the painter sitting across from you when she announces that she is bored by her own paintings? Can you feel what it is like to habitually need to do things in a meticulous way—to bind anxiety through vigilance and carefulness—and then to try to risk making a large mess by writing a novel? How high the stakes feel, though nothing more than putting words on paper is being ventured!

When I train creativity coaches, which I've been doing for twenty-five years, I ask them what "joining" means to them and when (and if) they've experienced it. Elizabeth, a coach-in-training, explained:

> As I thought about joining, with myself and with clients, I realized that the less I joined with myself, the less I was able to join with clients. I would do with clients what I did with myself: stand to the side, appraising, making assessments, and applying some arbitrary standards and, of course, more than a few "shoulds."
>
> What I've come to see is that when I step to the side like that (an excellent skill in some ways), somehow I abandon the meaning-making part of myself. Not only do I abandon that part, I also heap on it a lot of negative self-talk. When I do that to myself, I soon feel down and low energy because I've been berating myself inside without even registering it.

I like to use the word "partnership" to describe an inner connection where aspects of self can find a way to engage, dialogue, and have a give-and-take interaction instead of an "it's either you or me" kind of relationship. I think it would also help if I make it a goal to stop presuming and taking an attitude of superiority and laying down of "shoulds" toward myself and to find another place in myself (a fair-minded "overviewer") to look upon both "sides" with compassion and fairness. With that approach, I trust that I will end up taking my clients' side too, and join better with them.

At the heart of joining is a willingness to listen. There really is no substitute for deep listening. What we hear not only affects what we say but with how much emphasis we say it. For instance, we may hear a client saying that she wants to do X but that she also doesn't want to do X, for Y and Z reasons. In the split second of hearing this we make judgments as to whether Y and Z seem to us to be "good reasons" not to do X or "insufficient reasons" not to do X. We will push for X more or less strenuously according to our instant calculations. This is a natural result of us having been really listening.

The better we have heard our client on X, Y, and Z, the more appropriately we will respond. For example, I had a client who wanted to make certain anti-war sculptures for an upcoming museum exhibit but who also didn't want to create a stir in her small town with those anti-war sculptures. I wondered, should I more say to her, "Yes, I understand about not wanting to cause a stir" or "Go for it!"

My sense, as I listened to her, was that her own objections were very powerful and present and that she would ultimately want to shy away from the project. Therefore, I supported her in beginning her anti-war sculptures but I supported her with only modest energy. When she came back a month later to say that she really wanted to do something else, I wasn't surprised or disappointed and was ready to move with her in a new direction. I had "heard" her say this already in the previous session; this, now, was simply confirmation.

By listening, we hear the nuances. Having heard those nuances, we are much less surprised by whatever transpires and a much more skillful helper. Nor does this happen just once, somewhere in the first session. Rather, we join anew each time we interact with a client. One of the ways we accomplish this is by coming to each session with an empty mind or a clearing of the mind, so as to quiet our worries and be really ready to listen. This clearing of the mind is also a bit of personal good luck, because it means that there is nothing for you to be thinking about or trying to recall as you begin. The way to join is actually the easy way, which is kind of miraculous.

Maybe you have the feeling that you should clearly remember what you and your client talked about last time and that you should have prepared yourself in some way for the new session, as if there were some necessary homework that you should have engaged in between sessions. In fact, there is nothing much to remember and nothing much to prepare beyond recalling the basics of your game plan, if you are working with a game plan, and the details of any homework that the two of you agreed upon. You are remembering only a little; and emptying and being present a lot.

Each session is a new encounter. If your client has no particular place to begin, you can say, "Where did we leave off last time?" or "What's been on your mind?" We work in the present and if something doesn't come up here and now, there is probably no particular reason to dredge it up from your mental files or your memory banks. Of course, if you are monitoring an agreement ("I believe that you were going to make it to a twelve-step meeting every day last week?") or if you're in some other way obliged to remember something, that's one thing. But many sessions can simply begin with you saying, "What's on your mind today?" You let joining occur anew as your client starts speaking and as you start interacting in the present moment.

Whenever I come into a session with an idea, an intention, or some thought, I am much less present and do much poorer work. This runs entirely counter to what I believed as a young person, about having ideas, theories, and so on. Now I believe that our chief aim is to keep an "empty mind" as we listen, for two reasons: then we are really listening; and our whole brain is available to respond. If we breathe regularly and deeply (to counteract anxiety and to make sure that we are settled and present) and make sure that we are thinking nothing (except the thoughts that arise directly in conjunction with what our client is saying), we will do our best work.

Joining means inhabiting your client's universe and getting into her shoes. Joining, for a creativity coach, means understanding that a client who wishes to write as brilliantly as Shakespeare need not be expressing any unhealthy narcissism or unwarranted grandiosity but only high ideals and grand aspirations. Joining means understanding what a hundred consecutive rejections of a person's poem or short story does to the heart. Joining means understanding that the anxiety your client is presenting—her "artistic anxiety," if you like—is more like a ground of being, intrinsic to the struggle, than a symptom to be relieved.

Joining, for a creativity coach or anyone working with creative individuals, means letting go of theoretical or stereotypical thinking about creatives and learning about them by being with them. In walks a Jackson Pollock, a Virginia Woolf, a Vincent van Gogh, a Marilyn Monroe. In walks an extraordinary and well-defended creative person. For something good to happen, a creativity coach must smile and say hello and begin to join. This is not a ploy or mere technique on the creativity coach's part. Rather, it is a practiced and heartfelt way of opening the door to help and to change.

For any helper—coach, mental health counselor, family therapist, clinical psychologist, psychiatrist, etc.—you join by:

- Getting to know yourself: If you are shadowy and unknown to yourself, your client will feel like she is walking into a dark place.

- Calming down: The more anxious you are, the more your client will feel that she is a big problem to you and some sort of threat to you; and the more she will believe that you are unequal to the task of helping her.

- Listening: Clients know if you are listening or if you are just waiting for your turn to speak.

- Offering heartfelt support: A tiny bit of heartfelt support is more valuable than a mountain of rote support.

- Not presuming: You know lots of things and many of those things will help your client. But that is not the same as presuming that you are superior to him or her or that you can quickly know for sure what is going on in his or her mind or life.

- Being present: When something scares us in life (just as interacting with our clients may) we want to run away, fight back, or dodge the problem and rationalize away our inability to remain present.

Confronted by the scariness of a client with real challenges, pressing needs, abundant defenses, and quite possibly an array of demands, your goal, despite what may be your desire to flee, is nevertheless to stay present.

• Not thinking about you: You are not impervious to feeling hurt, challenged, criticized, or threatened by something your client says or does. It is certainly important that you protect yourself but it is also important that you do not overreact or grow too defensive when a client disagrees with you or isn't happy with something you said. Let your interactions be about your client and not about you.

To join means to take your client's side and to wish her well. Clients will intuit when you are holding that intention and they will intuit when you are not. You accomplish this by "being there." The essence of helping is not about doing but about being. A humane helper knows how to be with another person, how to sit quietly, how to accept another person's reality, how to tolerate another person's emotionality, how to hold a person's hand without literally holding it, and how to listen so that the person across from her feels heard and is heard.

It will naturally tax a humane helper if her client is talking a mile a minute, refusing to speak, describing the CIA's effort to spy on him or blaming everyone else for his difficulties. But even though taxed she will have trained herself to remain present, benevolent, and helpful. Whatever there might be for her to "do" at such times, her first and most important offering is the way that she is.

That way may be very active and involve a lot of leaning forward. "Being" doesn't imply passivity, silence, a lack of energy, or a lack of involvement. Robert Stolorow is the author of *World, Affectivity, Trauma: Heidegger and Post-Cartesian Psychoanalysis* and *Trauma and Human Existence: Autobiographical, Psychoanalytic, and Philosophical Reflections* and the coauthor of eight other books. He explained to me in an interview:

What is the proper therapeutic stance toward trauma and vulnerability? How can a therapeutic relationship be constituted wherein the therapist can serve as a relational home for unbearable emotional pain and existential vulnerability? Recently, I have been moving toward a more active, relationally engaged form of therapeutic comportment that I call emotional dwelling.

In dwelling, one does not merely seek empathically to understand the other's emotional pain from the other's perspective. One does that, but much more. In dwelling, one leans into the other's emotional pain and participates in it, perhaps with the aid of one's own analogous experiences of pain. I have found that this active, engaged, participatory comportment is especially important in the therapeutic approach to emotional trauma.

The language that one uses to address another's experience of emotional trauma meets the trauma head-on, articulating the unbearable and the unendurable, saying the unsayable, unmitigated by any efforts to soothe, comfort, encourage, or reassure—such efforts invariably being experienced by the other as a shunning or turning away from his or her traumatized state. Essentially, I am using myself to communicate to my client, "This is hard and here we are."

(Maisel, 2016b)

Or take Michael Cornwall's way of being. Michael has been available to individuals who are emotionally suffering for almost forty years, leading workshops at the Esalen Institute on compassionately being with people in extreme states while also writing for the Mad in America website. Michael explained to me in an interview:

From the time when I was slipping into madness in the 1970s until this second, I've never believed that such a shallow narrative as psychiatry has coughed up could ever in a million years explain what an overpowering, mysterious, and unbelievably shattering experience that my own madness journey was for me. So, I've never seen anyone else's emotional suffering of any kind through that distorted, untrue lens either.

I still spend every week in my office with people in extreme states who are taking or not taking meds. Imagine waiting, your heart harmlessly open and receptive to whatever emerges emotionally and energetically from another in their journey of madness or emotional suffering of any kind. That's the practice—being there, quiet when silence is wanted by the other, or engaged in a non-stop conversation if that's what they want.

An hour sometimes passes where I don't say a single word! My heart open, my tears falling if moved to tears, no cares interfering regarding diagnosis or theory or doing, doing, doing. Just being there with love. It's really that simple. If I had a loved one in emotional or mental distress, I'd try what I just described about listening while being receptively loving, while at the same time allowing oneself huge disbelief about what the disease model of psychiatry says is true.

(Maisel, 2016a)

As a humane helper, being with a person means all of the following:

Understanding what it means to be human. One example of understanding what it means to be human is remembering that an objectively small threat, like her in-laws coming to visit your client, might cause your client huge anxiety. It is not ridiculous, strange, or pathetic that the person sitting across from you can be made so agitated and upset by the prospect of such an "innocent" visit; an anxious reaction of that sort is completely common. This is just who we are: odd creatures who can bravely confront the enemy in battle and who can also feel woeful, embarrassed, and down-right frightened giving a two-minute speech at work, hosting a get-together, or having to fly across the country.

Striving to be her human best. Striving to be her human best involves exchanging her cynicism and misanthropy, qualities that exist in each of us, for feelings of compassion and respect for the person sitting across from her. It might be nice if she really felt that compassion and respect but whether or not she genuinely feels it, she nevertheless leads with it, just as a believer might "love her neighbor as herself" even if she didn't love her neighbor in the slightest. That is, she sets the bar in a high place, demanding of herself that she be respectful, warm, tolerant, and kind as she works with her clients.

Shifting from expert to investigator. A humane helper entered her helping profession for many reasons but no doubt among them was the desire to look like an expert, to be accorded the material and psychological perks that professionals receive, and to have her ego massaged by being called "doctor" or "counselor" or something similar. But she has to be wary of this desire, because wearing the mantle of expertise makes it very easy for her to act like she knows more than she in fact knows and to presume that she can accomplish more that she can actually accomplish.

A humane helper will want to shift her stance from "expert" to "investigator." This crucial shift is an internal one, away from acting like you know, a stance more appropriate for her plumber or her accountant, toward an attitude of experimentation, the stance of a scientific researcher involved in some serious investigations. That scientist knows lots of things and has all sorts of tactics and ideas and hypotheses; but he doesn't act like he knows the answers to his questions until (and only if) he really does know.

Marrying warmth and directness. Therapy outcome studies show that it is the quality of the relationship that best predicts a successful outcome and that the single most important element of that relationship is the warmth of the helper. Our humane helper is not a "cold" expert but a caring human being. Outcome studies also show, however, that an important predictor of a successful outcome is whether the client is engaged and "in it" with the helper. In order for this engagement to happen, our humane helper needs not only to demonstrate warmth but also directness. To this end, a question she might very well ask the person sitting across from her is, "Can we be honest?" She will almost certainly not ask it precisely that way: she will find her own language for saying this. But she will say it; because part of being present is not flinching and making sure that what needs to be said gets said.

Holding a large, broad view. Rather than narrowing her view, which the current mental disorder paradigm automatically does, our humane helper maintains the large, broad view that she is dealing with a complicated human being embedded in complex social, cultural, and political contexts who is not necessarily going to be that easy to read or that easy to help.

She therefore might begin each new encounter by murmuring, "I bet a lot is going on," allowing for the spaciousness of any sort of response her client would like to offer. In this calm way, she gets to learn a bit about how this individual organizes his reality, how his cultural background colors his beliefs and opinions, what he wants out of life, what he wants to avoid in life, and how he typically handles life's challenges. A feature of "being" is allowing for this sort of spacious responding.

Being human and being present aren't the same things as being self-revealing or sharing personal anecdotes. In my experience, the telling of such anecdotes usually deflects a helper and her client from the heart-to-heart work they were doing the minute before. It can be very useful for me to say to a writer client, "I was writing for more than twenty years before a major publisher signed me on." That helps anchor the idea of long apprenticeship, it never being too late, perseverance, and so on. But I think that to say more or to give additional details would prove unwise and deflecting.

Some humane helpers will feel that saying even that much is too much. Others will "use themselves" and their history freely in session. Revealing ought not to be forbidden and many humane helpers find it an integral and essential part of their work. I do think, however, that we have to be careful. Sometimes we "reveal" just because we are feeling anxious and don't know what to do or say next or we reveal because we want to paint ourselves as interesting, experienced or attractive. We may blurt out an anecdote or a piece of personal history so as to reduce the tension we're experiencing or because we feel some sudden desire to name-drop or experience-drop. Because we are tempted to act in such ways, it's important to carefully monitor our revealing.

Sometimes the hardest challenge we face as humane helpers is an inability to relax and communicate in a simple, human way with our clients. The tension produced from tightly holding worries like "What should I do next?", "What does all of this information I'm getting mean?", and "What will she think of my performance?" can easily get in the way of a helper sitting quietly, nodding, and responding. When a client comes to me, I really don't know what will work. I'm not worried that I don't know—indeed, I am very easy with not knowing. All I can do is relax and be human and be present.

That doesn't mean that, as humane helpers, we don't possess tactics, strategies, game plans, or ideas—that is, that we don't "do" things. We indeed do things. But it matters who we are and how we are. I am off on the wrong foot if I am just checking items off a checklist with an eye toward some diagnosis followed by a chemical fix. I am off on a second wrong foot if I take barely any interest in your story, your circumstances, and your concerns. And I have no leg to stand on if I am not present and unable to empathize with you.

POINTS FOR REFLECTION

1. What, if anything, gets in the way of you being present to another person? For any obstacle or impediment that you identify (for example, anxiety about not knowing what to say or what to do), explain how you might handle that obstacle or impediment.

2. Do you currently do a good job of listening to people? If you don't, what might you try to do in order to improve?

3. Picture yourself sitting across from someone who is talking a mile a minute or who has nothing to say. How does that make you feel?

4. Consider the idea of "joining with clients" (while still maintaining good boundaries). How would you describe this "joining" in your own words?

5. Consider the idea of "marrying warmth with directness." Describe in your own words how you might practice this.

REFERENCES

Maisel, E. (2016a). "Day 12: Michael Cornwall on Being Present to 'Madness.'" *Psychology Today*. www.psychologytoday.com/blog/rethinking-mental-health/201601/day-12-michael-cornwall-being-present-madness

Maisel, E. (2016b). "Robert Stolorow on Emotional Trauma and Psychoanalysis." *Psychology Today*. www.psychologytoday.com/blog/rethinking-mental-health/201602/robert-stolorow-emotional-trauma-and-psychoanalysis

6 Being with a Real Person

Humane helping is made much harder by virtue of the fact that human beings are not easy. They are not easy in many senses. Sometimes they are so disturbed and so out of control that you can't reason with them or communicate with them. Sometimes they are so sad, despairing, and defeated that they have virtually no energy left with which to help. When you take into account all of the ways that human beings can be disturbed, defensive, and difficult, it's unlikely that you'll ever see an "easy" client.

This shouldn't really surprise you. Just think of how hard it would prove to try to help your mother, father, brother, sister, or best friend actually change. Think of all of your own shadows, negative thoughts, defensive tactics, and unproductive behaviors. Are you easy? Almost certainly you aren't. So, if someone is coming in to see you and wanting a pill, wanting to blame his spouse, wanting to talk but not listen, wanting insights but not the subsequent work, wanting to get better but not to change, and so on, how surprising is that? And what sort of collaboration can occur in such circumstances?

How often are human beings really interested in reducing their emotional distress? Do they always or even often want to feel better? What if feeling better requires that they change their daily habits, change their habits of mind, change their circumstances, upgrade their personality, and work like the Dickens on every aspect of their life? How many people are up for tasks of that sort? It isn't just the person in some extreme state with a name like "schizophrenia" who is difficult to reach and difficult to help. It is each of us.

A given person may be suffering and may seek out a helping professional whom he hires to help relieve his emotional distress. Unfortunately for both the sufferer and that humane helper, he may nevertheless have powerful reasons for not cooperating with the person he has just hired. Maybe he doesn't want his drinking, smoking, or eating habits tampered with. Maybe he doesn't want to change—he wants the people around him to change. Maybe he's unwilling to reveal what's going on because he's embarrassed by his thoughts or by his actions. Maybe ... this list is very long.

If he is like this, that would make him entirely human and not very unusual. In fact, virtually all human beings prefer being who they are to being helped or to reducing their emotional distress—if being helped and reducing their distress make work for them, require that they change, or force them to look in the mirror. It looks to be an artifact of evolution that our "selfish genes" cause us to defend ourselves even against useful, life-improving help. It might be in a person's best interests to make certain admissions and take a certain amount of responsibility for his own self-care but most human natures rebel against this approach to life.

Taking all of this into consideration, where should we set the bar with respect to what we, as humane helpers, should reasonably expect of our fellow human beings? The experiments run by social psychologists suggest that we had better set the bar quite low. The many fascinating experiments of social psychology paint a picture of man as a thoughtless herd animal, as someone easy to manipulate, carelessly sadistic, and adamantly unaware. Milgram's famous learning experiments, for example, exposed human beings as creatures willing to deliver electroshock to their fellow creatures for no other reason than being told that they should. Zimbardo's equally famous prison experiments showed us how quickly average college students became sadistic prison guards or weak, frightened prisoners in virtually a matter of moments.

In Asch's well-known conformity experiments, in which subjects were asked about the lengths of lines, fully 75 percent of subjects announced that one line was the same length as another line, even though it transparently wasn't, just because others in the room said that it was. In Darley and Batson's Good Samaritan experiment, seminary students on the way to deliver a lecture on the importance of being a Good Samaritan could not be bothered to stop and help a person in distress. These and scores of other revealing experiments prove that the majority of human beings, and sometimes virtually everyone in a given experiment, seem incapable of thinking for themselves, acting in accordance with their professed values, withstanding peer pressure and other social pressures, or keeping their shadowy—and often barbaric—instincts at bay.

Therefore, why should we expect the average person to rise to the occasion and think clearly, courageously, and smartly about his own mental health or possess the wherewithal to dispute the current system of mental disorder labeling? Imagine if you ran an experiment designed to see how easily subjects embraced some new "mental disorder" label and, having embraced it, willingly began a regimen of chemicals to "treat their disorder." Let's picture that and predict the results. A doctor dressed in hospital garb comes in and explains that it has recently been discovered that boredom is a mental disorder. He gives it a fancy name and describes the symptoms of the disorder, symptoms chosen because all human beings experience them on occasion. He makes up some number—say, 75 percent—and claims that 75 percent of Americans suffer from this mental disorder and that a new drug is now available to treat it.

By the end of this experiment, how many people in that laboratory setting would agree that they had this mental disorder and would enthusiastically begin taking this "medicine"? Probably virtually everyone, if previous studies are any indication. It is a fair guess that a doctor dressed in hospital garb would be able to turn almost every subject into a "mental patient" with little or no effort. Would anyone raise an objection and exclaim, "Wait, boredom isn't a mental disorder! It's a natural reaction to something boring you! You shouldn't take a chemical to cure a lack of life purpose! What nonsense are you promoting here?" Would even one person in the room rise to make that speech or to voice some similar objection? Odds are that they wouldn't.

Would it matter if the room were filled with Bolivians, Japanese, Germans, or Americans? Probably not, since the experiments of social psychology are regularly run across cultures with identical results. Would it matter if the group were all men or all women or some combination of both? That probably wouldn't matter either. In all cultures where medicine is respected, it's a fair bet that folks in that room would open their mouths wide and start on a drug regimen for their newly diagnosed mental disorder.

A humane helper must deal with the shadowy nature of human beings, including their insatiable desire for chemicals. In a way, this makes it easier on her, as she can relax as she reduces her expectations. But of course, it also makes it much harder. Consider the reality of the thing we call "personality." The conserving nature of personality itself fights against our ability to act freely and improve our mental health. Because the conserving nature of personality maintains distress and because change is uncomfortable work, we should expect that a person who claims to want to feel less sad may well do surprisingly little to actually become less sad. This is exactly what we see.

In a model of personality that I've described elsewhere, of personality being comprised of original personality, formed personality, and available personality, the conserving nature of both original personality (our original endowments) and of formed personality (who we become over time) look to severely limit our available personality (our remaining freedom to be who we would actually like to be). This is true for everyone, which helps explain why change is generally and routinely difficult for human beings. The change might be as inconsequential as moving your bed slightly to the right or to the left: given the conserving nature of personality, even a minor change of this sort can feel daunting and dramatic.

The larger changes we've been discussing are that much more difficult to facilitate. It may seem odd to say that a person who is chronically sad remains chronically sad because of this creaturely inclination to conserve his formed sense of self—and yet that looks to be the case. It looks to be easier to stay sad than to become a different person. It looks to be easier to repeat your charges against the world than to stop bringing those charges. It looks to be easier to fear the same thing over and over again, even when it has proven no threat to you, than to stop fearing it. All human beings suffer from this same evolutionary disability.

Given these realities, what can a humane helper do? In other chapters, I discuss tactics like being present, creating game plans, working eclectically, and so on. Here I want to focus on what I think is an invaluable aid in reaching difficult people—that is, in reaching all human beings. It is a humane helper's practiced ability to speak directly to a person's "executive awareness," to that part of a person that is still free and able to hear, that is thoughtful, that operates according to values, and that would like its host to live a good life. I believe in this construct and use it in my work with clients.

"Executive awareness" is of course a metaphor, just as are "ego," "conscience," "the unconscious," and so on. For me, personally, it has a lot of utility and power. I have the feeling that I can actually speak to "a part" of the person sitting across from me that is his "best" part, his "most reasonable" part, his "least damaged" part, and his "still optimistic" part. To my mind, this executive awareness is the instrument of our available personality and of our existential intelligence and can be addressed and enlisted. When I work with a client, it is to that part of a client that I am speaking.

What does that speaking sound like? It sounds like the following:

"I want to speak to the part of you that knows best. Can I speak to that part?"

"Right now you're caught up in a lot of confusion. But you also have a lot of wisdom, don't you? Can we try to access some of that wisdom?"

"Every day we do some things that come from our shadowy self and some things that come from our best self. Which things come from your best self?"

"Something is seriously bothering you and you don't quite want to talk about it. All right. But isn't it the case that part of you knows that talking about it is absolutely necessary?"

"Tell me about the part of you that isn't at all happy with the choices you've made."

"I get it that your husband is impossible. But part of you must recognize the role you're playing in this dynamic?"

I find that I can go somewhere deep and useful very quickly by speaking in this way and by presuming that my client, as difficult as he may be, possesses this executive awareness and, if he is invited in the right way, can "step back," make use of this facility, and be more truthful, more helpful, and more present than he might otherwise have been. This way of operating is comprised of the language I use, the tone of voice I use, the way I hold myself, and the sense of safety and intimacy I create. This is all practiced; and this practiced way of being can aid a humane helper in working with even her most difficult clients.

Indeed, we might conceptualize part of our work as helping our clients increase their executive awareness. Let's say that a person is plagued by that combination of appetite, raw energy, desire, meaning crisis, pestering self-talk, and racing brain pressure that we nowadays typically and thoughtlessly label as "mania." What if increased executive awareness served both as a preventative, allowing an individual to notice that he was speeding up and giving him a chance to dispute his mania, and as an intervention in the moment, allowing him just enough space to keep his mania mediated rather than unmediated? We do not know if this is possible because we do not promote this ability. Who knows if increased executive awareness might not help prevent full-blown mania or other distressing states? And, since it just might, why not promote it as part of the work we do with clients?

Unless we posit some function like executive awareness, it's hard to see how a human being could know that he was stuck when he was stuck or how he could ever get unstuck. But because we do possess executive awareness, that ability to step aside and observe our formed ways of thinking and being, appraise them, and change our mind, we can not only change but even change in an instant. Maybe, as in the case of a drinking driver running his car into a tree, it will take a dire event for his executive awareness to kick in. But it can also happen in session effortlessly and instantaneously. By paying attention to this possibility and by speaking directly to that part of your client that is free, capable, and highest-minded, you give the two of you a chance for some rapid improvements.

If we can't manage to step back and employ our executive awareness, there is no distance between us and our stress, our painful feelings, our pestering thoughts, our rage, or our despair: we are glued to all that distress. Therefore, the cultivation of executive awareness might help across the board with regard to every so-called mental disorder; and this particular overseeing might amount to the very definition of mental health. This is another way of saying a commonplace but nevertheless important thing: that increased insight, increased awareness, and increased self-regulation are hallmarks of a healthy person.

A humane helper might say to the person sitting across from her, "If I can help you step back and get some space between you and the things that are bothering you, you might have a chance to come up with some new answers. Or at least a breath of fresh air might pass through you! Right now, your formed personality is a bit of a straitjacket, just as it is for everyone. Let's release the grip of that straitjacket as best we can. Do you want to give that a try?" Without ever mentioning executive aware-ness or any other concept or construct, you can begin to help your clients crack through their defensiveness and their denial and grapple with their complicated reality.

Whether or not you can reach this part of a person, enlist it, and make important, rapid progress, what you don't want to do is write off people, either consciously or unconsciously, because they are being difficult. Psychiatric survivors often report that, while they were unavailable to be helped during their most disturbed times, they nevertheless could sense and appreciate when a helper was trying to be of help and holding them as a worthwhile human being versus the more usual response to them as an inconvenience or a malignancy. Many report that this made a real difference to them and ultimately aided them in their recovery.

Even if two helpers are obliged to take the exact same action, say restrain a violent person in an in-patient setting, it still matters to the person being restrained if one helper is restraining him compassionately, as it were, and if the other is restraining him as if he were a dog. As humane helpers, we must remember this. Even if we can't reach a client, even if we are frustrated by a client, even if we have rather little hope for our species or for individual members of our species, our goal still remains to be of help and to not dismiss other human beings.

The current, dominant paradigm and its labeling system provides for the subtle or gross dismissal of people by virtue of labeling them personality disordered, schizophrenic, and so forth. The current chemical dispensing program has the same effect. It is a variation of dismissal to act as if providing a chemical is an answer to life's challenges. Because it looks pseudo-scientific and pseudo-medical, it is somehow easy to swallow the idea that providing a label and a chemical amount to our best standard of care. But it is actually a form of dismissal. Humane helpers, who recognize that all human beings are difficult and that disturbed and distressed individuals may prove more difficult than average, must do more than this.

The current thrust of mental health services provision in the direction of "diagnosing and treating mental disorders" and "medicating patients" is rooted in large measure in this reality, that helpers must try to help individuals who aren't easy and who aren't helping much. What psychia-trist isn't much happier acting like you "have something" and writing you a prescription than trying to arm-wrestle you out of your personality, your habits of mind, and your ways of being? Wouldn't you be rather likely to do exactly the same thing in his position? And yet we mustn't. If we are championing humane helping, we must refrain from too-easy solutions.

It may be that, as my client, you are more unwilling to cooperate, say because you have secrets to keep, or it may be that you are more unable to cooperate, say because your chronic sadness has drained you of the energy you need to collaborate. These are different situations but from a helper's point of view they amount to the same problem: you aren't helping. And that likely will have consequences for you if you happen to visit a traditional helper working according to the dominant paradigm, where your lack of cooperation will get factored into the diagnostic label you get and, in turn, into your prognosis and your treatment plan.

Say that you are uncooperative and maybe even loud about it, perhaps in part because you have some intuitive sense that you are not going to get the help you need. The more difficult you are, the less likely you are to get some "mild" adjustment disorder diagnosis or some "mild" mood disorder diagnosis and the more likely you are to get a "severe" personality disorder diagnosis or some other "severe" diagnosis. Just as a judge has a remedy for "difficult and unpleasant" where he works— namely, his power to hold you in contempt—a helper-as-judge has his remedy as well: the ability to diagnose you with a "borderline personality disorder" or an "oppositional defiant personality disorder" or something else that translates as, "Wow, you are very difficult!"

Of course, this is a covert and maybe even only a half-conscious operation. A psychiatrist would never say to you, "Because you are being uncooperative I am going to give you a harsher label." Nevertheless, he is indeed likely to provide you with that harsher diagnosis, and for two different reasons: because he is annoyed with you but also because once he gives you that pejorative label he is relatively off the hook as far as treating you goes. Since it is "well known" that folks with personality disorders are by-and-large unreachable and untreatable, his job has just become that much easier. A person's unwillingness to participate in reducing his own emotional distress coupled with a helper's wish to make it easy on himself when dealing with uncooperative clients leads us to this exact moment in the history of mental health, where chemicals are running rampant and everyone acts as if human beings have caught various versions of some mental flu.

It also follows that the more difficult you are, the more society will react coercively. Produce headaches for your parents and psychiatrists are waiting. The more antisocial you act the more society will want you handled. Your screaming on the street will not be tolerated. Your suicide gesture will be criminalized. Society wants peace and quiet. Why should society's desire to protect itself surprise anyone? If you throw your pumpkin soup in the face of your waitress because you believe that she is trying to poison you, society cares about only one thing: you must stop that.

Where we have arrived, then, is the completely predictable result of two agendas marrying: the marriage of the sufferer's wish to remain the same and the helper's wish to make it through the day. We must somehow factor this reality into the way we as humane helpers operate. A humane helper will be faced with this intractable reality however she manages to do her work. She should expect a client to be bound up in his personality and rather straitjacketed by it. She should expect him to be rather a herd animal and so insufficiently practiced in self-awareness as to have only limited executive awareness available to him. She should expect only a marginal level of cooperation from him, because of human defensiveness, because change is difficult, because we who claim to help may not be seen as trustworthy, and so on. Because she is not naive, she understands all this.

Still, even very difficult people—the most distressed, disturbed, and defended among us—can change, heal, make progress, recover, and in other ways seriously improve. Sometimes this change can occur in an instant, whether it's by driving into a tree and "hitting bottom" or, more propitiously, by interacting with a humane helper in some meaningful way that turns out to make all the difference in that sufferer's life. Both realities are true: that human beings are difficult and that humane helpers can nevertheless serve them, sometimes beautifully and quickly.

You might suppose that a difficult human being could not be helped that quickly or that beautifully, given a whole lifetime of him being adamantly himself. But it happens all the time. That is important to remember. You may not experience this great good luck with any given client—but you will experience it with some clients, even with many of them. The more practiced you get at speaking directly to that part of each human being that is still able to listen, the more often you will get these excellent results. You can look forward to this!

POINTS FOR REFLECTION

1. Think of the "normal" people you know. How easy or hard would it be for any one of them to make a significant personality change?

2. If people are likely to remain themselves (through the conserving nature of personality), how must that influence humane helping?

3. Translate the phrase "executive awareness" into your own language. Is this a concept or metaphor that you might profitably use?

4. Imagine that a person has "just so much" available personality (or freedom) with which to gain insight, make changes, and reduce his distress. How might you access that available personality?

5. On balance, does understanding that human beings are essentially difficult free you up to relax or make you more anxious?

7 Where Will You Focus?

Where will you focus as you work with the person sitting across from you and as you try to help him? You might, as your starting point, decide to "just be" with your client and let him lead and direct the work. But in the course of your work together you may decide that he is not seeing something important that he ought to know about and so you may want to alert him to your point of view. That is, sometimes, and perhaps much of the time, your client will take the lead and sometimes you will take the lead. However, even if your client is technically leading, it is still you who is deciding. Helping is about "being there" but it is also about you deciding where you intend to focus.

Where might you focus in your work with a client? The following sixteen areas (among many other possible choices) are reasonable places to focus:

1. You might focus on what your client asks you to focus on.

2. You might focus on what you think it is important to focus on.

3. You might focus in areas where your training or theoretical orientation suggests that you focus.

4. You might focus on matters that you are mandated to focus on.

5. You might focus where your client believes you will focus.

6. You might focus on trying to understand what is going on.

7. You might focus on some short-term goal or objective.

8. You might focus on some long-term goal or objective.

9. You might focus on explaining something to your client.

10. You might focus on skill building or habit building.

11. You might focus on your client's circumstances.

12. You might focus on some matter that spontaneously arises.

13. You might focus on your game plan.

14. You might focus on safety, either yours or your client's.

15. You might wonder aloud, "What should we look at next?"

16. You might "just be there."

Let's look at these sixteen in turn:

You might focus on what your client asks you to focus on. Your client has things on his mind. If he came in to see you of his own accord, he can probably say at least in a tentative way why he came to see you. He may report in a global way, for example, "Everything is a mess"; he may report in a way that echoes the dominant paradigm, for example, "I think I'm bipolar"; he may report in a way that is customarily taken to be a symptomatic way, for example, "I've lost all interest in everything"; or he may report in some other of the countless ways that human beings express what's distressing them. One way or another, he is likely to want to tell you what's on his mind—and that's where you can focus.

If your client hasn't come in of his own accord, if he has little to say and seems disinterested in being there, or if he's saying lots of words but not really identifying issues, that doesn't mean that he doesn't have things on his mind. In due course, if you can hang in with him and gain his trust, even a coerced client, a court-referred client, a disturbed client, a defensive client, or a reluctant client is likely to announce that something nameable is bothering him. That's where you might then focus.

This focusing can sound as simple as, "You say everything's a mess. Can you tell me a little more about that?" It can sound like reframing disorder language into the sort of language you want to use, for example, "You say you're bipolar? You mean that there are times when you're racing along and then there are times when you're sad?" It can sound like a beginning investigation of cause and effect, for example, "You say that you've lost interest in all your usual pursuits. Why do you think that is?" Your client presents something and you may well decide to focus your attention there in simple, human, common sense ways.

You might focus on what you think it is important to focus on. Your client may be unwilling or unable to talk about those matters that you think might be important for the two of you to talk about. She may wave off her self-starvation, cutting behaviors, or other self-harming activities as of no interest to her. But, of course, they may be of great interest to you. She may deny that her husband's extramarital affairs are bothering her, she may dismiss as so very long ago and of no current moment the way that she was humiliated in childhood, she may reject as unimportant your concern about her inability to sleep. But all of these may strike you as relevant.

As a humane helper, you do not simply nod and agree with your client when she waves off an issue. That is no more humane than, for example, agreeing with a wounded soldier that you should leave him to his significant injuries and go help his wounded comrade who is injured somewhere else on the battlefield. People have all sorts of reasons for steering you away from what is actually bothering them and what actually matters to them; therefore, you will need to learn your own diplomatic and effective ways of saying, "No, I think we'll stay right here." You mustn't be afraid to focus where, in your opinion, you think you ought to focus.

You might focus in areas where your training or theoretical orientation suggests that you focus. I'll present the case in a later chapter for taking an eclectic stance as a helper rather than relying too dogmatically on the theoretical orientation in which you were trained. But that isn't to say that you might not want to employ those elements of your theoretical orientation that you like, that you believe in, and that you think really do help.

For instance, if you're a cognitive-behavioral therapist, you would logically and properly focus on your client's self-talk. If you're a meaning coach (a specialty I'll describe further on), you would logically and properly focus on your client's meaning challenges and life purpose choices. If you're an addictions specialist, you would logically and properly focus on your client's compulsive and addictive behaviors. That isn't to say that you wouldn't focus in other areas, too. But it makes sense that if you have a specialty or a particular orientation and that specialty or orientation is an appropriate lens through which to view some portion of your client's reality, you would focus in exactly that way.

You might focus on matters that you are mandated to focus on. If you're working with court-appointed "drinking drivers," you may have to administer breathalyzer tests as part of your work. If you're working with self-harming teenage girls in an in-patient setting, you may have to check for sharp objects or check to see if they are cutting themselves. If you're working in an out-patient setting with teenagers starving themselves, you may have to weigh them. If you're working in virtually any setting and you are licensed in a traditional way, you will need to focus on reporting child abuse, elder abuse, and many other reportable issues should they arise.

Your focus must move from wherever it was to a clear, careful focus on mandated matters, since your job, your license, and your client's welfare and the welfare of others depend on you focusing there. Sometimes this shift in focus will only require a brief detour and sometimes it will shift everything, for instance if you have to hospitalize your rail-thin client or report to the court that your "drinking driver" client is coming to sessions intoxicated. Whether these detours are brief or protracted, they are mandatory.

You might focus where your client believes that you will focus. It may be the case that over time you have shifted your practices away from your theoretical orientation and away from allegiance to the dominant paradigms and toward a more eclectic approach that hardly resembles the way you first worked as a less experienced helper. But your client may believe that you are still working in that former way, perhaps because you still call yourself a Freudian analyst, a cognitive-behavioral therapist, or a psychiatrist. If your client is expecting you to work in a certain way, you will need to focus there at least long enough to explain to your client how you now work.

For example, as a cognitive-behavioral therapist you might say, "We're going to pay a lot of attention to the way your self-talk may not be serving you and may be promoting your anxiety and your unhappiness. That's really important work. But we'll also be looking at any traumas you may have suffered, because I've learned over time that looking at only your self-talk and your current behaviors isn't quite enough. Does that make sense to you?" In this way, you reassure your client that you will be focusing on matters he presumed you'd be focusing on while expanding the playing field to include other ways of helping that you deem useful.

You might focus on trying to understand what is going on. A question our humane helper asks the person sitting across from her is, "How should we think about this?" She is making her guesses and coming to her conclusions and at the same time she is inviting the person sitting across from her to think about his situation, come up with his own suggestions and conclusions, and be "in it" with her.

For example, a humane helper might say, "You say that you have no trouble paying attention to the things that interest you but that you have terrible trouble paying attention at work and to things your wife says to you. How should we think about that?" Then she pauses and waits. She gives the person sitting across from her a chance to actually think about that. She provides a "space" and an "opening" for him to mull her words over and chew on them. With luck, he will have some ideas and will share those ideas with her and the process will continue in this richly collaborative fashion.

You might focus on some short-term goal or objective. A question a humane helper might ask the person sitting across from her, maybe even virtually every time they chat, is "What sort of work do you want to accomplish during the coming week?" or "What do you want to focus on between now and the next time we chat?" One of her tactics can be to help her client name short-term goals and other short-term efforts. Our current forms of helping typically do not include a focus of nameable short-term goals but a humane helper might well want to incorporate this active and direct way of working into her practice.

For example, she might get in the habit of summarizing at the end of a session in the following way: "Okay, we've decided that you'll try three things this week to help you shake your sadness. One, you'll get out every day and walk—no days where you stay inside all day please! Two, you'll either think about drafting that letter to your parents about all the things you want to get off your chest or maybe you'll actually draft it. Three— and I know this is the hardest—you'll reach out to that fellow you mentioned and set up a coffee date, even though that feels really, really hard. Okay?" By operating in these sorts of ways, a humane helper helps her client know exactly what they are working on in the short term.

You might focus on some long-term goal or objective. A question our humane helper can ask the person sitting across from her is, "What do you want us to keep in mind over the next few months?" or "What do you want to try between now and the end of the year?" or some variation on the theme of long-term focus. She then checks in on these long-term objectives and co-creates new objectives if her first formulations turn out to be not quite right or not quite working. She helps her client keep track of these long-term goals and monitors the roiling that will doubtless go on in her client's psyche as he tries to live purposefully and intentionally.

For an anxious performer, for example, a long-term goal might be mastering one or two anxiety-management skills and practicing them in real-life performance situations. For an alcoholic businessman who is fighting with his wife, avoiding home, and neglecting his children, the marriage of a short-term goal and a long-term goal might be going directly to an Alcoholics Anonymous (AA) meeting after work every day and then going directly home to spend time with his wife and children—and doing that for the next six months straight. For a sad, lonely college student, a combination of ongoing goals and long-terms goals might be involving herself in her college's peer counseling program, spending less time in bed and more time outdoors, and coming to some hard but necessary conclusions about whether her current major holds any passion or even any interest for her.

You might focus on explaining something to your client. Helping can include explaining and teaching. If you're a creativity coach, as I am, you might explain the benefits of a morning creativity practice, the nature of everyday resistance to creating, and some tactics for cracking through that everyday resistance, and why completing creative projects can prove so maddeningly difficult. You might teach a client about the idea of "triggers" and help him identify which specific triggers precede his binge drinking. You might do some teaching and explaining in any number of areas that arise spontaneously as the two of you work together.

You would likely not stop and deliver a full lecture at such times. But if a moment arose when providing a simple explanation seemed useful, you would do exactly that. Over time you might get very practiced at delivering certain explanations in a concise way that served your clients without disrupting a session's flow. In some models of psychotherapy such explaining and teaching are roundly condemned; but they can prove excellent tactics as part of our more humane model.

You might focus on skill building or habit building. Reducing our distress often requires that we acquire a new skill or habit. It may take news skills for us to adequately deal with being bullied, avoid our drug-using friends when we are trying not to use, or live independently from our toxic family. We may need to acquire the habit of asking for what we want, refusing to give away our time to anyone who asks for it, or shutting the bedroom door when we need some peace and quiet. As a feature of upgrading our personality, an upgrade that virtually all of us might benefit from, there are doubtless new skills and new habits that would be worth acquiring.

A humane helper might begin by explaining that a new habit or a new skill takes time to put into place, that her client can expect setbacks along the way, and that if he experiences a setback he should forgive himself instantly and just as quickly recommit to practicing the habit or skill. A humane helper can, if the following method feels congenial to her, describe the skill or the habit, invite her client to customize it, and then from session to session monitor her client's progress in acquiring the skill or habit. This is a simple, useful place to focus.

You might focus on your client's circumstances. We'll chat about the importance of circumstances in a future chapter. Circumstances matter; circumstances create stress and distress; a radical change in circumstance or even a certain small change in circumstances may make all the difference as to whether or not your client can actually reduce his distress. Here let me underline one feature of circumstance. A humane helper may well want to pay much more attention than she currently does to the role of socioeconomic conditions and social and cultural realities in the lives of the clients she sees.

Living in poverty matters; being a member of a marginalized group matters; dealing with a strict, rule-bound extended family matters; feeling endangered in your own neighborhood matters; facing limited prospects by virtue of the circumstances of your birth matters. The power of society to exert control and to inflict emotional distress also matters, for example when it labels a person for life with a mental disorder label. If, for example, her society asserts that refusing to "medicate" a rambunctious child is tantamount to child endangerment, then anyone who disagrees with that vision, whether helper, parent, or child, will find themselves on a collision course with the powers that be. This all matters and can legitimately be a focus of your work together.

You might focus on some matter that spontaneously arises. In the course of chatting about his history of nightmares, your client might say, "I had that particular nightmare when I was in boarding school." That bit of new information may strike you as something to file away and not focus on; or it might strike you as something worth investigating right on the spot. You might inquire as to whether he thinks chatting about his boarding-school experiences would be worth some of your time together; if he shakes his head you can resume where you were and if he nods his head you can ask a question like, "Tell me a little bit about your time there."

Whether you spend time on those experiences or not, having given him the chance to chat about them will please your client, who will recognize that you were listening, that you have the common sense to know that boarding-school experiences can be traumatic and influential, and that you had no "pushy" or voyeuristic agenda around forcing him to talk about those experiences. Having stopped for a moment in that way, as simple as that was, will impress your client, cause him to trust you more, and further build the helping relationship.

You might focus on your game plan. You may decide to create a game plan (which in the pseudo-medical language of the current dominant paradigm would be called a "treatment plan"), refer to it, and keep to it so long as it serves you. We'll discuss this in detail in a subsequent chapter and follow that discussion with an examination of a "life formulation" model that is one specific sort of game plan. Here the idea to underline is that you may well decide outside of session where you want to focus in session. The other places to focus that we've been chatting about are related by virtue of the fact that they are decisions that you make in session. But you might also make some decisions outside of session and then bring them to session.

For example, say that an element of your game plan with a given client was your desire to have him reduce his reliance on smoking cigarettes as his primary way of managing his anxiety. You might come into session with that agenda item in mind and announce, "I'd like us to begin by focusing on your smoking. You mentioned a while ago that you'd like to stop smoking and we haven't chatted about that much because we've been looking at other things. Can we focus a bit on the smoking today?" If he agrees, then you might proceed in any one of many sorts of ways, for example by asking the simple question, "What might you do instead of smoking when you're feeling anxious?" Shortly we'll look at this idea of game-planning more closely.

You might focus on safety, either yours or your client's. Sometimes you must focus on protecting yourself from your client, protecting your client from himself, or protecting others from your client. Your client is abundantly human, which means that he can become violent toward you, suicidal or self-harming, or a threat to others. Whether you drive a taxi, run a bakery, or sit in a comfortable office, anyone who deals with other human beings has to be careful. You have to be extra careful, for three reasons: your license, if you are licensed, will come with legal obligations regarding your reporting duties; you are working with people already in distress; and your work with people already in distress may prove provocative.

You might wonder aloud, "What should we look at next?" A question our humane helper may sometimes ask the person sitting across from her is, "What should we look at next?" Maybe the two of them have come to completion during a session on a given issue. Her client knows what his marching orders are: he knows what he is going to try during the coming week and why he is trying it. Our humane helper is likely quite aware that other things are also going on in his life and now might be a moment when she turns to one or another of those other things.

She could be quite directive and say, "Shall we look at the following next?" Or she could ask, "What should we take a look at next?" Either is a plausible way to continue helping. A third, more elaborate way to proceed is to say, "We've been looking at a, b, c, and d over these last several weeks [maybe his drinking, his relationship issues, his unhappiness at work, and his general sadness]. We just came to some nice closure on 'a' for today. Shall we perhaps look at b, c, or d now?"

This is an excellent approach, if a humane helper can pull it off, because it provides a kind of running summary of the work that she and her client are engaged in and provides a menu from which her client can choose the next issue to tackle. Whatever specific approach a humane helper takes in this regard, one of her basic approaches can be to ask as is needed, "What should we look at next?"

You might "just be there." The simplest, most humane, and most helpful place to focus is on being present. Your client is a person who needs you not to be thinking about your unpaid bills, your too-busy day, your children's antics, your theories about human nature, your desire to try out some strategy or tactic, or your worries about whether you know enough to be of help or can stand listening to the problems of yet another person. Your client needs you to be present, available, thoughtful, compassionate, unafraid, and helpful.

If you are present you will make connections among the many things your client has to say, understand the weight of his challenges and the constrictions produced by his formed personality, feel his anxieties, disappointments, and regrets, and be able to gauge in a tentative way what is possible for him to try, whether that is a lot or a little. You'll begin to nod and ask questions and wonder aloud and press here and there and sigh with him and maybe begin to paint a picture of what he might want to try in order to reduce his distress and improve his lot. You may find that you are doing this rather effortlessly, since "just being present" is really a kind of ease rather than a kind of work.

Of course, it isn't the case that you switch your focus during session in some formal, mechanical way, as if you were switching gears while driving. Rather, you have these many ways of operating available to you and you avoid the temptation of believing that there is only one right way to operate and only one place worth your attention. With your child, you might play with her on the floor one moment, get up and begin her dinner the next, and struggle with her to get her teeth brushed after dinner; and one might conceptualize these transitions as different areas of focus or just what parenting looks like. Likewise, one might conceptualize the above sixteen as different areas of focus or just what helping looks like.

POINTS FOR REFLECTION

1. Consider the sixteen areas of focus discussed in this chapter. Which seem the most congenial to you and the places you're most likely to focus?

2. Which of these sixteen seem the least congenial to you? Why do you suppose that's the case?

3. Do you like the idea of focusing on short-term goals and objectives? If you do, how might you incorporate that focus into your practice?

4. Do you like the idea of focusing on long-term goals and objectives? If you do, how might you incorporate that focus into your practice?

5. In what other areas not covered in this chapter might you focus?

8 Creating Game Plans and Inviting Homework

Imagine that you are sitting with a dear friend who is listening to you describe your current despair. She might say very little or even nothing; she might or might not offer any suggestions; what she almost certainly wouldn't have is a prepared "game plan" for helping you. Nor is it likely that she would try to improvise one on the spot. Yet without anything like a game plan, or what in the mental health field, using inappropriate medical model language, is called a treatment plan, she might still prove to be of great help to you, just by virtue of being there in a certain way.

What you, the sufferer, may want at that moment is a shoulder to lean on, a human presence, an attentive ear, and, yes, some wisdom and maybe some useful suggestions. But do you need a complete, full-blown, detailed game plan from your friend? No. Your friend need provide no such thing to still be of great help. Likewise, a humane helper can be of help in exactly the same way just by being human, by listening, by nodding, by being present, by giving you the chance to express yourself and hear yourself think out loud, and, yes, by offering thoughtful suggestions too. Her suggestions do not amount to anything like a game plan; and they may be enough.

However, she can go a step further and also game plan; and, as part of her game planning, she might invite her clients to engage in homework. Just as a football coach both creates game plans and also spells out to his players what they should practice in the week before the game, a humane helper can include "practice" as part of her game plans. A coach explains to his quarterback that he had better get his passes off quickly because the opposing team has a fierce pass rush and orders his quarterback to practice quick release during the practices leading up the game. A helper can do exactly the same thing: she can co-create a game plan with the help of her client and co-create the activities that her client might try between sessions to "put the game plan into action."

To continue the football analogy, if you are playing football you know clearly what you are trying to do: score more points than you allow. To do that you create a specific game plan based on the skill set of your players, your opposition's tendencies, and so on. As easy as that is to understand, coaches vary tremendously in their ability to game plan well. One coach gets the most out of his players; another gets much less. One coach has an uncanny ability to call the right play at the right moment; another coach seems regularly to call the wrong play.

We would expect helpers to fall along a similar continuum. If game-planning is not your long suit, then in order to add game-planning to your repertoire you will need to practice and become more proficient. One way to practice is to prepare a "life formulation write-up" for each of your clients, as described in the next chapter. By creating such a written document you'll have helped yourself to think about who your client is, what she's presenting as her concerns and which additional or different concerns you have, what your hopes are for her, and what your suggestions will be, including your suggestions for homework. In medical lingo, this would be called a treatment plan. Since what a humane helper is doing is nothing medical, it's more appropriate to call it game planning than treatment planning.

"Game plan" in a humane helper's context might mean any of the following. It might mean that since her client is presenting "excessive drinking" as an issue, she will use ideas and language from the twelve-step recovery movement in her work with this client. It might mean that, since her client keeps returning to the theme of "not knowing what my life is about," she will present him with a picture of "life purpose choosing" that includes explaining how he can create a menu of life purpose choices, try each out experimentally, and see which seem the richest. It might mean that, since the teenage boy sitting across from her seems only to like video games and nothing else about life, she will use the language of video games and chat about "meeting the challenges at each level of the game." And so on.

Then, like a football coach who creates an elaborate game plan during the week before the game but is obliged to chuck it out the window if a blizzard suddenly strikes at game time, a humane helper might create a game plan for a given client but still retains the flexibility to shift her focus and her energy depending on what is actually going on in session and in her client's life. If sadness is suddenly the issue, then sadness is suddenly the issue. If marital discord is suddenly the issue, then marital discord is suddenly the issue. If an emotional blizzard strikes, that is her new reality. A humane helper learns over time how to do both: co-create a game plan with her client's assistance and update her game plan in the spur of the moment.

In a given extended interaction with a client, one that may take the whole time you have together (that is, the whole session, if you are working a session model), you and your client may find yourselves chatting about something that does not seem directly related to the issues you've identified or that in fact isn't related to those issues but represents another challenge that your client is facing. Spending your time in this way is not a violation of some abstract rule about "keeping to the game plan" but rather an acknowledgment that game planning is not a strict or limiting activity but instead a gentle roadmap for helping. If today you and your client take some detour, who is to say that it's a detour?

Say, for example, you're chatting with someone who has come to see you because she is in despair. Maybe for the first time in session it comes up that she never had children because her husband never wanted them. She explains to you that she in fact wanted them but deferred to her husband's wishes. Now, in her early forties, there is a slim possibility that, with some heroic measures, she could still perhaps get pregnant. That issue is now squarely on the table and it would make little sense to go "somewhere else" just because you'd had a plan for the session or because you were working from a game plan.

You know from your life experiences and your understanding of human reality that this must be a complex, painful subject and that your client probably had her own reasons for not having children separate from her husband's reasons. Therefore, you might be tempted to skip chatting about this subject because you want to avoid something so charged, complicated, and shadowy. Still, you know that you really ought to stay present and not run away from this authentic issue. This chat was certainly not part of your game plan and you may not love the idea of having to engage in it, but you do—because you want to be of help.

Out loud, you might say, "How should we hold this?" or "Is this part of what's making you sad?" or "Tell me more." You invite a continuation.

Your client may well have no answers and may want to stop talking about this painful subject, one that may be laced with guilt and self-recriminations. If she wants to stop, do you stop? Because you have a game plan, you might nod, let the subject close of its own accord, and move on to something else that the two of you are working on. Or you might decide to stay put and continue investigating, calculating that the pain that this conversation might bring is really nothing compared to the pain that your client might experience if she moves past her childbearing years not having fully resolved this issue. Which is the right way? It is impossible to know for sure. Having a game plan doesn't rescue us from the reality of not knowing which is the wiser approach.

However, though they don't rescue us from that reality, game plans nevertheless serve an excellent purpose. They remind us where we intend to focus, help us keep our client's long-term goals in mind, and aid us in understanding whether or not some progress is being made. As discussed in the last chapter, you might focus in any one or several of a great many directions as you try to be of help; and having so many directions available can feel daunting. A game plan is a way to organize those many possibilities.

Remember that you are not treatment planning, as if you were doing medicine. A treatment plan has about it the idea that there is one right way or only a few right ways to approach a problem—a cast put on a certain way and worn for two months (or maybe a sling instead), followed by physical therapy performed a certain way for the next two months (or maybe three months, depending on your progress). To be sure, treatment plans are not necessarily rock solid, especially if the diagnosis is still up in the air. But game plans in a humane helping context have about them even less of a sense of assurance. A game plan is more a set of working hypotheses put into action, tested without guarantees in the crucible of reality, and altered according to the results you see.

And what about assigning homework as part of your game planning? What are your thoughts on that helping activity? If your preferred style is to be present, to listen, to lean forward, to nod, to acknowledge what your client is feeling, to reflect back what your client is saying, and so on, do you also need to make suggestions that amount to assigning homework? Is assigning homework more a matter of personal choice and a stylistic matter or is it perhaps so important a part of "what helps" that it really ought to be embraced by every helper?

My personal opinion is that educating a client that "work" will be needed and aiding that client in designing that work are crucial and not incidental parts of the helping process. I think it is wise and humane for every helper, mental health professionals of course included, to actively wear a so-to-speak coaching hat, especially at the end of a session, and discuss goals, suggest homework, and monitor any homework that might be assigned.

"Homework" just means inviting and assigning a concrete task, one that both of you understand and agree upon. This might be as small as getting out in the sun three times in the coming week or as large as beginning to think about a new profession or beginning to disengage from a toxic relationship. Of course, these invitations are not offered from on high, as if you and only you know what might amount to sensible homework for your client. Rather, a humane helper asks the person sitting across from her questions of the following sort: "What do you think we should try?" or "Given what we've been talking about, what do you think you might like to try this coming week?"

A question of this sort doesn't come out of the blue but is a natural thing for a helper to ask in the context of the conversation that she and her client have been having. For example:

Helper: Tell me more about the bullying.

Distressed teen: It's been getting worse since I cut my hair! Now they're calling me a dyke!

H: Is the bullying exclusively name-calling? Or do they do other things too?

DT: They do lots of things. Pushing me. Knocking things out of my hands.

H: I'm curious. Can you think of one thing to try in the coming week that might make things better? I'm curious if anything comes to mind.

DT: Like what?

H: I don't know. I was just wondering if anything came to mind for you. If not, no problem! But take a moment and see if anything comes to mind.

If nothing comes to your client's mind, you simply continue in whatever way you might continue next. But if something does come to her mind, you might profitably "stay there" and patiently, gently, and carefully see if her insights lead to some nameable work. You might help her refine the nameable work so that it is more doable, help her visualize actually doing it, help her strategize as to when she might do it and under what circumstances she might do it, and so on. At the end of a conversation of this sort your client would possess an excellent idea of what she might try during the coming week to deal with the bullying she's experiencing.

Or you might, for example, offer an anxious client three or four anxiety-management strategies to choose from and suggest that he try out one of them during the coming week. You might wonder aloud with your blocked creative client whether he might want to start his day creating, rather than waiting for the evening when he is tired and defeated, and, if that seems like a good idea, whether he might like to try to do that this coming week. You might propose to a client struggling with life purpose and meaning issues that she spend time during the week "creating a list of possible life purpose choices" or "creating a list of possible meaning opportunities." And so on.

In my opinion it is a good idea that a humane helper asks her client to do things, in addition to and often rather than just talk about things or think about things. Whatever the size of the thing that she suggests that he do—whether she suggests that he "take a small step" this week or "take a big risk" this week—she does not leave him without things to try. She doesn't say, "Let's keep talking about this next week." What she says is, "I look forward to hearing how trying that out went." Her client may have gained some important insights during the session; but then there ought to follow some useful work between sessions.

As a humane helper, you might build a repertoire of homework assignments that you discover through practice and experience regularly serves people. For instance, with many clients and with regard to many diverse issues, you might invite a client to monitor her self-talk in the coming week and notice if and when she says things to herself that don't particularly serve her. You might ask many of your clients to practice an anxiety-management technique, a stress-management technique, or a mindfulness technique, or work on a certain communication skill like speaking without apologizing or speaking without criticizing. Who wouldn't benefit from this work?

A humane helper might also invite, help co-create, or offer very specific assignments that flow from her particular work with a given client and that flow from the guesses she makes as to what might potentially help that client. For example, say that her client is sad about his inability to find meaningful work. Say also that the helper remembers that her client mentioned a few weeks before that he once truly loved dinosaurs. She might "out of the blue," but nevertheless completely in context, suggest the following homework assignment: "You know, I wonder what it would be like for you to visit our natural history museum and wander among the dinosaurs. Care to do that this coming weekend?"

She doesn't have to have a clear idea as to why she is bringing this up. She may merely have a feeling or an intuition. If her client responds, "No, I don't think that connects to anything," she might nod and say, "All right. Let's pick up where we left off." If her client responds, "I think I'd love to do that," there's nothing more that needs be said, except perhaps, "Which day of the weekend do you think you might like to visit the museum?", thus helping her client make the task more concrete. If he says, "Saturday, I think," she can simply continue with, "Great! Let's see what comes of that!"

It is of course too coercive and dictatorial to say, "You must do this!" to clients. But it is humane and compassionate to say, "So, are we agreed that you'll try this in the coming week?" You smile a warm smile that reads, "We have some hope, yes?" and "Good luck to you!" No frowns; no demands; no suspicious looks; no subtle declarations of defeat. Just a kind-hearted "You'll give this a try, yes?" and "Who knows, something good might come of this!"

OVERCOMING YOUR RELUCTANCE TO ASSIGN HOMEWORK

If you're currently reluctant to assign homework, maybe because it runs counter to what you've been taught or counter to some tenet of your theoretical orientation, but you nonetheless think that assigning homework might be a good idea, here are some possible counters to the reluctance you may be feeling. Check if your reluctance is on the following list; if it is, see if the counter I provide helps you dispute and dispel your reluctance.

Reluctance: "I don't like being pushy."

Counter: "I'm not being pushy, I'm being inviting."

Reluctance: "I wouldn't know what to assign."

Counter: "I can play it by ear and see what my client thinks."

Reluctance: "What if it doesn't work?"

Counter: "That's nothing like a tragedy; and at a minimum it will be a good learning experience for both of us."

Reluctance: "What if my client doesn't do the homework?"

Counter: "I'll be easy with that, I won't overtly or subtly guilt-trip him about that, and we'll chat about the experience to see what we might learn from it."

Reluctance: "Assigning homework doesn't match what I was trained to do."

Counter: "Experience is the best guide and if experience is telling me that assigning homework is a good thing, let me try it."

Reluctance: "My theoretical orientation rejects the idea of directive interventions and explicitly warns against assigning homework."

Counter: "I can't be slavishly attached to theory; I have to learn from my actual practice."

Reluctance: "The clients I work with are so disturbed or disengaged that assigning them homework makes no sense."

Counter: "I might still try to find an appropriate small thing for even my disturbed and disengaged clients to try, on the grounds that you can't know for sure what might reach a disturbed or disengaged human being."

Inviting homework is not a magic bullet or a gold standard. It is simply a reasonable, human, and humane thing to try with a client with whom it makes sense to try.

If you are trying to help someone who is very stubborn and who is not only clearly unwilling to work but is not even slightly willing to chat about working, inviting homework would not be high on your list of tactics to try (though it might still be on that list somewhere). Likewise, if you're attempting to help someone who is filled with despair and who can barely make himself stay alive, a conversation about homework, no matter how heartfelt or humane, would almost certainly fall on deaf ears (though you never know). With some clients, today may not be the day to try to assign homework. But with a great many it just might be.

You invite homework because you believe, suspect, or hope that doing a particular thing will help your client. But which particular thing might you suggest? Well, first, you would invite your client to see what he thinks might make sense as homework. Say, however, that nothing comes to mind and it looks to be on your shoulders to make a suggestion. What might you suggest? That depends in large measure on how you're conceptualizing what's challenging him and what might help with that challenge.

For example, say that you are helping a despairing, hard-drinking out-of-work man in his late forties who lives on his own in a not-so-good neighborhood and who is complaining that he can't sleep, that he can't find work, that he's tired all the time, that his back hurts, and that his life is mess. Were you to focus on his drinking, you might suggest that as homework he attend an AA meeting. Were you to focus on his job difficulties, you might suggest that as homework he visit a certain jobs office that you know about. Were you to focus on his sleep difficulties, you might suggest that as homework he change his sleep routine in a particular way. Were you to focus on his fatigue or his back problems, you might suggest that as homework that he get a complete physical, if he could afford that; and if he couldn't, you might point him in the direction of a free clinic. Were you to focus on his despair, you might suggest that as homework he do one thing in the coming week that might make him feel a little more hopeful about life, say visit his granddaughter and play with her a bit. Each of these is a reasonable invitation and represents an honorable attempt to help.

The particular suggestion or suggestions you make are based on your understanding of what helps human beings and on the specifics of your work with this client. You can't ask your client to do everything "at once" and you can't know which is the "very best" homework to suggest. What you can do is relax, surrender to the truth that he can only be expected to do so much, and make a simple suggestion or two based on your sense of what might prove beneficial to him.

Of course, you could present him with many options and ask him to choose; and a limited version of that approach, where you make three or four suggestions and invite him to choose one or two, might prove quite useful. But even there you are choosing which three or four to put on the table. Whenever you make a suggestion of any sort, you are deciding where you want to focus. Relax with that truth, that you are aiming clients in a given direction by virtue of the decisions you make, and invite the homework that you think is sensible to invite.

Inviting homework is no more arcane or complicated a process than what I've just described. A person is sitting across from you; many things are challenging her; if she seems like a candidate for homework, you ask her what she would like to try in the coming week; if she comes up with something, that is her homework. If she can't come up with anything, you make suggestions based on your understanding of what might possibly help. You do this because you believe that human beings are helped when they are invited to try out real things in the real world. You don't overburden a client with homework; but by the same token you don't underestimate what a client might be ready and willing to do.

POINTS FOR REFLECTION

1. Describe in your own words the difference between a game plan and a treatment plan.

2. Do you see yourself as more of a "being there" sort of helper or a "game planning" sort of helper?

3. If you can see the virtues of being both, how might you balance or integrate those two different attitudes and energies?

4. If you can see yourself giving homework, what sorts of assignments might you give?

5. What do you see as the upside and the downside of game-planning?

9 Experimenting with Formulation

In the last chapter, we looked at the idea of creating and updating game plans and inviting homework. One well-known game-planning procedure practiced in psychotherapeutic circles, especially in the UK, is what's called formulation. A helper thinks about the person she's helping and formulates her thoughts, often in a narrative way by writing out what her client is presenting, what she, the helper, thinks is going on, and what she thinks might help. She is asking herself and trying to answer two specific questions: "What's going on?" and "What might help?"

A question our humane helper asks herself and also asks the person sitting across from her is, "What's going on?" By asking the question this specific way, she means to not narrow her client's responses and to not "pull" for any particular kind of response. "How are you feeling?" pulls for a "feeling" response, "What's bothering you?" pulls for a "I'm bothered by" response, and so on. "What's going on?" allows the person sitting across from her to start in any way that he likes, whether that's to complain about his job, wonder aloud about "the meaninglessness of it all," pick a "symptom" to underline (like sleeplessness, inattentiveness, etc.), or even scratch his head and say, "I don't know exactly."

The person sitting across from our humane helper explains what's going on as best he can. As he shares his thoughts and feelings and begins to explain himself and his situation, our humane helper begins to hypothesize herself about what's going on. She begins to formulate her opinions, guesses, hunches, and intuitions, which then leads her to her next steps, to the suggestions she makes and to the further clarifying questions she asks. In operating this way, she is neither diagnosing, as if something medical were going on, nor hunting for some label to attach to her client. She is just gathering her thoughts and deciding how to proceed.

In this ordinary, everyday, human-sized interaction no "diagnosing" need go on. The straightforward alternative to "diagnosing" is not diagnosing and having a human interaction instead. When there are countless possible causes of a thing like a smile or a sigh, we can either lump everyone who smiles together and lump everyone who sighs together, creating categories of "people who smile" and "people who sigh," or we can create a million individual "categories" for each person who smiles and for each person who sighs. Neither activity makes sense or is worth the effort. Rather, we sit with a person, think about that particular person, and wonder both internally and aloud about how to proceed.

Imagine that a given person is sad because he has no life purpose, another person is sad because his best friend is doing better than he is, a third person is sad because his mate is cheating on him, a fourth person is sad because he can't get over his childhood abuse, a fifth person is sad because he hates his government's policies, a sixth person is sad because winter has lasted eight months, a seventh person is sad because he can't get his novel written, an eighth person is sad because she has become invisible to men, a ninth person is sad because he can't find the wherewithal to announce his sexual orientation, and so on.

The "naming" alternatives here are to create the category of "sad people" (which is what we currently do by turning "sad" into the "mental disorder of depression") or to make all of the following categories: "people who are sad because their novel isn't working," "people who are sad because their mate is cheating on them," and so on. Is either naming operation useful or sensible? Is it useful to lump all sad people together under one umbrella? Likewise, would it be sensible to create a million categories of sad people based on our guesses about what is making them sad? What would be the point to either naming operation?

Consider a second example. Imagine several unruly boys at a school. One is unruly because he is bored, a second is unruly because he is being picked on, a third is unruly because his parents fight all the time, a fourth is unruly to gain attention, a fifth is unruly because he's already a mean son-of-a-gun, a sixth is unruly because he finds math hard, and so on. To repeat, we can only do one of three things here with respect to naming. We can pin a single label on all these boys, using words like "defiant" or "oppositional" or "attention deficit disordered," and claim that they all have the same "mental disorder." Or we can create a separate category for each "type of unruliness." Or, most sensibly, we can admit that these boys really have nothing particular in common except an observable behavior. Either we create an empty category, endless categories, or no categories at all. Only the latter is honest.

Taxonomies of convenience are not legitimate. Each person is his own story. No theory about him is true; no category into which you put him is a legitimate definition of him. This is the high ideal at the center of humanistic, existential, and person-centered therapy, that each person should be considered a person, acknowledged as a person, and accepted as a person. What flows from this way of thinking? One possibility is that you sit there, chat with your client, and organize your thoughts about him or her. A version of this organizing is called "psychological formulation."

Psychological formulation has a long history and if you'd like to read up on it I suggest that you start with Lucy Johnstone and Rudi Dallos's book *Formulation in Psychology and Psychotherapy.*

LUCY JOHNSTONE ON FORMULATION

Dr. Lucy Johnstone is a consultant clinical psychologist, author, lecturer, and trainer. She was lead author for the British Psychological Society's Division of Clinical Psychology "Good Practice Guidelines on the Use of Psychological Formulation" (2011), author of *Users and Abusers of Psychiatry* (2000), and co-editor of *Formulation in Psychology and Psychotherapy* (2013). Her most recent book is *A Straight Talking Guide to Psychiatric Diagnosis* (2015). The following is from an interview I conducted with her (2016):

Eric Maisel: You are involved in efforts to help practitioners better understand and better employ "psychological formulation." Can you tell us a little bit about what psychological formulation is and why you consider it useful?

Lucy Johnstone: The process of labeling someone's problems as an illness, or in other words diagnosing them, is the cornerstone of psychiatric practice. We urgently need alternatives, and in essence, all alternatives consist of ways of listening to people's life stories. Psychological formulation is one way of doing this, although not the only way. However, it has a firm foothold in UK mental health practice.

Briefly, it is the process of making sense of a person's difficulties in the context of their relationships, social circumstances, life events, and the sense that they have made of them. It is a bit like a personal narrative that a psychologist or other professional draws up with an individual and, in some cases, their family and the people who care for them.

The professional contributes their clinical experience and their knowledge of the evidence—for example, about the impact of trauma. The client or service user brings their personal experience and the sense they have made of it. The end result of putting these two essential aspects together, in written or diagrammatic form, is called a formulation. Unlike diagnosis, this is not about making an expert judgment. It is a shared, evolving, collaborative process which also includes the person's strengths, and which suggests the best route toward recovery.

Eric Maisel: How do you personally work with individuals in distress? What is your approach and what are your methods?

Lucy Johnstone: It goes without saying that formulation is at the heart of my clinical practice. This is true both at a one-to-one level and in the form of consultation known as Team Formulation, in which I facilitate meetings to enable a group or team of mental health professionals to develop a shared psychosocial understanding of a client's difficulties.

Since formulation is a kind of overarching structure for tailoring our knowledge and evidence to the individual, it is compatible with a number of different therapeutic approaches. I believe that all formulations should be "trauma-informed"—in other words, be based on an awareness of the prevalence of all varieties of trauma and adversity and the impact they can have on people's mental health. Therapy isn't the only way forward, though, and team formulation plans often highlight the need to work with practical issues about employment, benefits, and so on as the main priority.

What follows is my version of formulation, what I'm calling a "life formulation" model, which pays a lot of attention to the practical challenges that human beings face and makes a bright line distinction between the client's concerns and the helper's concerns.

In my life formulation model a humane helper would think about her relationship with her client in the following seven ways: 1) her client's expressed concerns; 2) her client's circumstances of note; 3) her client's behavioral and emotional considerations; 4) her client's life purposes, goals, and aspirations; 5) her client's challenges as inferred by the helper; 6) the helper's concerns; and 7) the helper's recommendations. There would be no DSM language or pseudo-medical language used in this model, no new diagnostic language would be introduced, and everything would be described in "plain English" (or plain French or plain German).

How might this work in practice? Let's consider a fifteen-year-old girl named Jane who is "brought in" to a helper by her parents. They believe that Jane is "depressed"; they are also worried about her drinking, her insomnia, her school difficulties, her thinness, and the fact that she is cutting herself.

First our humane helper would check in with Jane about Jane's expressed concerns. These might turn out to be that Mary likes Elizabeth better than she likes Jane; that the clique that includes Mary and Elizabeth will not let Jane in; that Billy prefers Elizabeth to Jane; that Mrs. Williams in English may well be giving Jane a C, ruining Jane's chances of getting into the college she is dreaming of attending; and that her parents are driving her crazy by always scrutinizing her and criticizing her.

There is absolutely no reason why these concerns can't also come with some sort of number, if that were deemed useful: it would not be hard to create a huge list of concerns and attach a number to each one, if that was wanted. In addition to the words describing Jane's concerns, there could also be numbers: let's say 1104, 1931, 2242, 4482, and 5561. It would be child's play to list those five numbers in a "summary report," if a helper needed to do such a thing. This would look like: Expressed Concerns (1104, 1931, 2242, 4482, 5561). (But I think there is a better way to do this summarizing: see later.)

Next would come an acknowledgment and understanding of Jane's circumstances, gleaned from Jane and maybe from the reports of others. This might sound like:

Circumstances of note:

- In Jane's family, a college education and a professional career are required.

- In Jane's family, it is not permitted to date someone from a different cultural or religious background.

- Jane is not permitted to lock her door or any door, including the bathroom door.

- Jane surprised herself by doing much more poorly in freshman year than she had expected to do.

- Jane's older sisters were the stars of her high school.

Are these all the circumstances one might include? Of course, they aren't. Are these the most pertinent circumstances to include? Who knows? But each is suggestive and each helps a humane helper understand Jane's reality. They may not be exactly the correct circumstances to note or a sufficient number of circumstances to note but they are important and they matter.

Next would come behavioral and emotional considerations. In Jane's case this might look like the following:

- Jane is cutting herself (confirmed by Jane).

- Jane is drinking excessively (disputed by Jane).

- Jane is quite sad (confirmed by Jane).

- Jane is starving herself (disputed by Jane).

- Jane is sleeping very little (confirmed by Jane).

Next would come an investigation of Jane's life purposes, dreams, goals, aspirations, and other existential and motivational factors. These could be reported in ordinary language and might sound like the following:

- Jane remembers her camp counseling experiences as particularly meaningful.

- Jane considers that one of her life purposes is to marry and raise a family although she believes that she would be a "bad parent."

- Jane would like to leave her small town and live in London or Paris.

- Jane sees herself as both "secular" and "spiritual" and would like to find a "spiritual outlet."

- Jane does not believe that she has any real chance to succeed.

Next would come inferred challenges, that is, the helper's ideas about what is going on. This might sound like the following:

- predictable challenges of adolescent girls in Jane's cultural and socioeconomic situation;

- special challenges of living in a strict, punitive family;

- emotional challenges of intense sadness and constant worry;

- cognitive challenges of self-denigrating and punitive self-talk;

- behavioral challenges of cutting, drinking, starvation, and sleeplessness.

These inferred challenges would be described in the helper's preferred language: the language of psychological formulation, the language of narrative psychology, the language of cognitive behavioral therapy (CBT), the language of Jung, the language of Freud or contemporary psychoanalysis, the language of existential psychotherapy, in "ordinary" or "everyday" language, and so on.

A helper could use whatever language she wanted to use, making sure to indicate where her language came from: that is, in addition to a long list of everyday inferences (like "the predictable challenges of adolescence") there might be also long lists of Jungian inferences, existential inferences, and so on. If a code was needed, coded items might appear as J462 for "Jungian mid-life crisis" or F993 for "Freudian arrested development in the anal stage" and so on. Hopefully these taxonomical niceties would not be needed or wanted. But if they were, they could easily be accommodated.

Next would come the helper's concerns. These would be expressed in ordinary language in the following sort of way:

- concerned that Jane has no one to talk to, given that she's on the outs with her successful siblings and that she has no confidante in either of her parents;

- wondering if Jane was born a little sad and, if so, if sadness will constitute a lifelong challenge for her;

- some suspicions of childhood sexual abuse given Jane's particular presentation;

- want to really focus on the sleeplessness and its causes, as sleeplessness can drive "mania" and "psychosis";

- must tackle the cutting, the drinking, and the self-starvation.

Next would come the helper's recommendations. This might sound like:

- cognitive work around self-esteem;

- depth work around possible trauma;

- behavioral work around eating, cutting, and drinking;

- behavioral work around sleeping;

- family work around expectations.

This represents the life formulation model in a nutshell. Let's take a closer look at some of its pluses. Some virtues of this life formulation model (and its accompanying life formulation guide, if one were constructed) include the following:

It not only avoids the word "diagnosis" and the very idea of "diagnosis" (and essentially ends diagnosing) but it also avoids the word "psychological" and announces that a humane helper is helping people in distress with their problems with living and not exclusively with their "psyche." Thus, for example, both "getting a job" and the "psychological consequences of not having a job" become legitimate areas of exploration.

A helper could as legitimately work on "job skills" or "social skills" as work on any traditional "psychological" or "psychotherapeutic" issue.

It doesn't conflate or confuse the person's concerns with the helper's concerns. Jane may not be concerned about her lack of sleep, her drinking, her cutting or her eating habits but our humane helper may well be. This model allows both sorts of concerns to find a place in the conversation and a way to get both sorts of concerns communicated to third parties.

It allows for conversations about, and reporting on, both "causes" (like suspected sexual abuse) and "treatment recommendations" (like, for example, cognitive work on self-esteem or behavioral work on stopping the cutting). No two helpers might look at "causes" or "treatment recommendations" in the same way but the life formulation model at least has built-in places for both to appear. "Causes" can appear in both "inferred challenges" and "helper's concerns" and "treatment" has a dedicated home in "helper's recommendations" (with the pseudo-medical word "treatment" studiously avoided).

Some items could so-to-speak "auto-fill." If, for example, it is generally accepted that everyone should have a complete medical work-up to see if the concerns presented are organic or biological in nature—to see, that is, if any "real" disease or medical condition is present—then one "standard recommendation" that could "auto-fill" would be "It is suggested that Jane have a complete medical work-up."

Likewise, if it is generally accepted that it is good to have someone to talk to about things, then the recommendation that "Jane should have the chance to talk in an ongoing way with a helper" might auto-fill. This latter point might seem obvious and might seem to go without saying, yet in the pseudo-medical model that I'm disputing it is not at all clear that "talking to someone" is seen as valuable, not when chemicals can be dispensed in a minute and save psychiatrists so much time and idle chit-chat. If a humane helper believes that "talking to someone" matters, it could be regularly included in her recommendations.

It allows for an interesting "tag" system of reporting. This is an important point. When you search for something on the Internet you introduce certain words or "tags" that help you find what you are looking for: say "solar system," "planet," and "rings" if you are looking for a planet with rings. This gets you to "Saturn."

Tags are not labels but instead are our attempts to partially describe an entity. You can partially describe a thing in a "list sort of way" by identifying its parts: legs, head, tail, and so on (this is "defining by denotation"). You can also partially describe a thing in an "idea sort of way" through the use of concepts: a horse is a carbon-based living creature descended from some now extinct other carbon-based living creatures (this is "defining by connotation").

Such describing and defining is always incomplete, imperfect, and more arbitrary than we would like to admit. We know from philosophers of language like Wittgenstein that every abstract word (say "war" or "love") has no real definition but rather a huge range of meanings and colorations. Maybe World War II is the exemplary or paradigmatic instance of "war" but it is not meaningless or inappropriate to talk about "the war between the sexes" or "corporate warfare." The same is true of words like ego, dysfunction, abuse, or any other abstract word that can be used to describe human beings, human behaviors, and human situations.

Tags "merely" help describe: they do not amount to a "diagnosis" and they do not pretend to present an exhaustive, complete, or even adequate picture of a life. That is a good thing, because we should be tired by now of all that pretension. In Jane's case, you could report on Jane by providing some number of items in the six categories—say five items per category—and produce a one-page report that is thirty lines in length. That is one kind of "description of Jane's situation." But you could also choose from among those various items and select some number of tags—let's say seven—that together provide a kind of snapshot of Jane's current reality.

For example, one helper might choose as her seven tags for Jane and her situation "strict and punitive family dynamics," "low self-esteem coupled with high expectations," "adolescence," "self-starvation," "sadness," "excessive drinking," and "cutting." Naturally each of these tags could come as a number rather than as words, if that was wanted. This snapshot would in no way provide a complete picture of Jane's current reality but it would do a more sensible and humane job than labeling Jane with a pseudo-medical "clinical depression" diagnosis and some additional "adjustment disorder" or "personality disorder" diagnosis.

What might this tag system sound like in practice? For one client, and according to one helper, the seven tags might be, "sad; unemployed;

mid-life crisis; recently divorced; health issues; 'addicted' to porn; no goals or aspirations." For another client, and according to another helper, the seven tags might be, "traumatic childhood; issues with food; dramatic relationships; spiritual seeker; creatively unfulfilled; uninspiring day job; lives in 'chaos and confusion.'" These snapshots could be created around any agreed-upon number of tags: three tags, five tags, seven tags, ten tags, and so on. The more tags, the more cumbersome the system but also the more complete the snapshot.

If you decide to set the bar as, "We need one word like 'depression' to capture everything that we need to know about a person's distress and his or her current situation," a tag system does not reach that absurd height. But if you decide to set the bar differently as, "We need a way of communicating a snapshot of a person's reality that includes some important features of a person's life and aims a helper in the direction of helping," a tag system would meet that threshold beautifully.

This model would "force" a helper to inquire about Jane's actual concerns, learn about Jane's actual circumstances, acquire a picture of Jane's behaviors, thoughts, and feelings, come to some conclusions about Jane's situation, and offer up some recommendations as to what might help. This would naturally improve service. Helpers would become smarter about human nature and about human challenges by virtue of having to think about how "cause and effect" operates in the lives of real people and having to consider what actually works to reduce distress. This model stretches and tests helpers in a useful way.

To be clear, as we are not always so clear about this, this life formulation model is not an alternative system of diagnosis but an alternative system to diagnosis. It allows for helpers to chat with one another, either through summary reports or a tag system, and if it were widely accepted it would force those entities that believe they need diagnoses (like, for example, the courts) to begin to change their mind. The courts and other institutions would be forced to accept that "hearing voices," for example, is a reportable thing but does not lead to some made-up "diagnostic label" like "schizophrenia." It would serve our vital communications needs and at the same time it would act as an agent of change.

No doubt other alternative systems to diagnosis can be dreamed up and one or another of them might provide even more pluses than this life formulation model. But this is a good start, I think; it could be enacted right now; and were it enacted it would revolutionize how helpers think about and care for the people who come to them in difficulty and distress.

This life formulation model would go a long way toward providing a helper with a conceptual framework that honors the richness of life and the naturalness of distress, and an organizational scheme that allows her to report in an honest way on a sufferer's experience. A model that by its very nature disputes the DSM and the ICD, that aids a helper in asking the right questions, and that distinguishes her concerns from her client's concerns might well prove extremely valuable.

POINTS FOR REFLECTION

1. Describe the idea of "formulation" in your own words.

2. How would you describe the difference between "psychological formulation" and "life formulation"?

3. What do you see as the value or virtue of a system like "life formulation" that allows you to make a distinction between your client's concerns and your concerns?

4. How might you integrate the idea of "formulation" with your theoretical orientation?

5. How might you use "formulation" in your practice?

REFERENCE

Maisel, E. (2016). "Day 13: Lucy Johnstone on Psychological Formulation." *Psychology Today*. www.psychologytoday.com/blog/rethinking-mental-health/201601/day-13-lucy-johnstone-psychological-formulation

10 Including Life Purpose and Meaning

The helping professions—all of them, psychiatry, psychotherapy, family therapy, coaching, etc.—have handcuffed themselves in their ability to be of enough help to the people they see by virtue of never having acquired useful, on-point language regarding our human needs for meaning and life purpose. Even existential psychotherapy and existential coaching, and sub-branches of these like logotherapy, which ought to have created good language to help individuals with their life purpose challenges and meaning issues, haven't.

This creates a huge hole in helping that needs plugging and that you can help begin to plug in your own practice. If the person sitting across from you isn't helped to understand the nature of meaning (as a certain kind of psychological experience) and the nature of life purpose (as something to decide upon, as in "These are my life purpose choices," as opposed to something to seek or find, as in "What is the purpose of life?"), your client is much less likely to significantly reduce her experience of distress. If her life purpose and meaning challenges remain, so will her distress.

How will this distress manifest? To take one example, many people spend their lives in a manic search for meaning or in a manic flight from the experience of meaninglessness without ever understanding that meaning isn't something that can be chased down and without understanding that fleeing the experience of meaninglessness only increases that experience. Much of what is causing "bipolar disorder" is likely this agitated search for something that will make life feel meaningful and help a person deal with the common experience, routinely felt by intelligent, sensitive people (exactly the sort of person coming into a psychotherapist's office), that life is "just not meaningful enough."

Sometimes a client knows that he is experiencing these challenges and can express his difficulties. Here is a portion of an email sent to me by someone in this sort of existential distress:[1]

Dear Dr. Maisel:

I am twenty-seven and male. My mental health history is long and complex so I'll summarize it by saying that I was diagnosed with ADHD as a kid and took Ritalin until around the age of eleven. I was then diagnosed with depression and anxiety and placed on Paxil, which gave me the symptoms of bipolar disorder that I was subsequently diagnosed with and for which I was treated for years. All of these treatments made me increasingly sick and unmotivated.

I finally went off all medication before I started college (around age eighteen), and eventually ended up at a university where I studied and had a decent time other than a couple of serious life crises and occasional bouts of depression and anxiety. I graduated with highest honors and a very good GPA, but by the time I graduated I was beginning a depressed episode that would be nearly continuous from the age of twenty-two until the present. I started smoking marijuana to cope with severe anxiety and depression around that time and have done so on and off since then.

I have almost no contact with the outside world other than occasional shallow conversations with neighbors (which I dread) and seeing my therapist once a week, but she isn't helpful and is mostly grounded in a form of Buddhist psychology I find very vacuous and unappealing. If I start talking about the meaning of life, she says things like "But don't you want to be happy?" as if I'm being a jerk by worrying about something as insubstantial as "meaning."

Everything in life feels like a chore. There is nothing I can imagine doing for long enough to make money from it. Occasionally I will get extremely interested in a subject or project, which has always been the case throughout my life, but instead of lasting for months like these interests used to, I become disenchanted and bored within a day or at most a week. After that I can't even force myself to engage with that topic anymore without feeling severely depressed. I've tried to get a job but anxiety, aversion, disinterest, and a sense of pointlessness just hammer me to the ground every time something comes up.

I feel like I've squandered my life away and like I don't even deserve to feel better or have anything good come from life because I have no talents, no skills, and nothing that makes me special other than this grinding depression. Most recently I traveled to a foreign country using some of the last of my savings, hoping for some kind of epiphany or change of heart. Instead I just felt incredibly alone and realized the emptiness even of beautiful beaches and the warm sun. It all just felt like it was being wasted on me, a piece of garbage with no hope for a decent life.

I'm contacting you because I've read parts of some of your books. I've tried to follow the programs in them but got stuck early on. I just haven't been able to come up with any meaning that could possibly apply to my own life. I have nothing to offer and I don't want anything particular from the world, so the obstacles I come up against immediately frustrate me to the point of complete apathy. I'm only writing this email because I'm desperate, but I have no idea what I'm desperate for. Maybe to feel like less of a loser and to think that maybe I'm worth something.

To this I replied (in part):

Well, you are at a good age to make some new meaning investments <smile>. As you probably know very well but perhaps need to remind yourself, you will have no life purposes until you choose your life purposes and little sense of meaningfulness until you make decisions about what meaning investments you want to make and what meaning opportunities you want to seize.

You ought not to expect life to "feel" meaningful—you have to dig into your values and principles and decide what sort of life would make you proud—that is, you must manifest your values and principles and, if you are lucky, experience life as meaningful as a result of having made those efforts. You have to muster the energy and the inner resources to TRY some prospective meaning opportunities to see if they in fact pan out. Meaning opportunities come with no guarantees. They are absurd, optimistic, hopeful guesses about what might existentially work.

Volunteer for something, write something, relate to someone, start juggling in public, do something completely different, try something—basing your guesses on the values and the principles you want to uphold. Make your life count by TRYING something—only then will you be able to see if that something "mattered enough." Yes, you have tried this before—and you must try it again. Create a new list of meaning opportunities—that's step one. Then DO some of them—that's step two. Good luck to you!

He responded (in part), "Thank you. I will give this a try. It actually helps a little to realize that there is no other option."

Did this small interchange turn his life around? Who knows? But isn't it interesting that he found even this minimal interaction helpful? What if a humane helper worked with him in the areas of value, life purpose, and meaning? What if that—and not his putative "mental disorders"—were the focus of the work? Isn't it just possible, bordering on quite likely, that such a focus would do more for him than more pills or new pills?

Humane helping includes dealing with the life purpose and meaning needs of clients. This work helps a client deal with current distress; it may also forestall future distress. What if some major future difficulties, like those events and states currently called psychosis and schizophrenia, could be warded off by helping individuals deal with their life purpose and meaning challenges sooner rather than later? This isn't an odd or preposterous idea, given the research indicating that psychosis may be a particular way of handling existential challenges. Paris Williams, one such researcher, explained on his blog for the Mad in America website:

While I don't believe it's a stretch to say that our attempt to validate the brain disease theory of these disorders has so far been a colossal failure, there is a very different line of research that I believe has had much more success in providing significant clues as to the cause of these vexing disorders. The line of research I'm referring to is the research that has inquired directly into the actual lived experiences of those who have personally experienced psychosis.

My own recent research is particularly relevant in this regard, which includes a series of three studies inquiring deeply into the experiences of those who have experienced full and lasting recovery from long-term psychosis ... I have found that the findings of this line of research have converged sharply upon a fundamental cause of these psychotic disorders that is perhaps best stated something like this: The individual we deem "schizophrenic" or "psychotic" is merely caught in a profound wrestling match with the very same core existential dilemmas with which we all must struggle. In other words, it appears likely that psychosis is not caused by a disease of the brain but is rather the manifestation of a mind deeply entangled within the fundamental dilemmas of existence.

... As the individual enters into a psychotic process, we can say that their very self, right down to the most fundamental levels of their being, undergoes a process of profound disintegration; and as we have seen in the recovery research, with the proper conditions and support, there is every possibility of their continuing on to profound reintegration and eventual reemergence as a renewed self in a significantly changed and more resourced state than that which existed prior to the psychosis.

(Williams, 2012)

Not everyone who experiences "psychosis" or "schizophrenia" comes out the other side in such good shape. It's likely that most don't, especially in a culture like ours that treats these events as medical phenomena and rushes to provide chemicals. Therefore, wouldn't it be nice to help your client not go through this process at all? Chatting with a person about his or her meaning and life purpose needs may help with his or her current distress. But just as importantly that conversation may also forestall future distress and may provide a client with other ways to deal with his or her existential crises rather than via psychosis or some other dramatic or disabling way.

Most helpers, humane or otherwise, haven't a clue about how to talk about life purpose and meaning with their clients or how to help sufferers deal with their life purpose issues and meaning crises. I hope that humane helpers will try and ultimately will become adept at helping the people they see articulate and live their life purpose choices and make and maintain meaning. One of the great blessings that a humane helper can bestow upon the person sitting across from her is getting his vague, unaddressed but keenly felt life purpose and meaning needs "on the table," where they can be aired, understood, and finally addressed.

Currently helpers tend not to take a client's meaning needs, life purpose concerns, or conflicts of values into account. How often do you suppose a client is asked, "Tell me a little bit about your life purpose choices and decisions" or "Are you more a meaning-maker or more a meaning-seeker?" The answer must surely be virtually never. These sorts of questions are not part of the everyday landscape that mental health service providers inhabit or part of either dominant paradigm, the primary "diagnose and treat mental disorders, usually with chemicals" paradigm or the secondary "expert talk/psychological issues" paradigm.

Such conversations are not so difficult to have. It is really not so hard to paint a picture of what value-based meaning making might look like, what it would feel like to make daily meaning investments and seize daily meaning opportunities, what it would take for a client to create his or her personal menu and mix of meaning opportunities, and what the process looks like for naming and framing a client's life purposes. The main problem is not the difficulty of articulating these concepts or the difficulty of translating these concepts into tactics and strategies but the fact that these matters are not on the radar of mental health service providers.

What might this work look like? Humane helpers, in addition to speaking in a language that promotes a focus on life purpose, meaning, and value, might also suggest all sorts of tactics that help the people they work with identify their life purposes, live their life purposes, create meaning, maintain meaning, and get their values and principles onto their daily to-do lists. We need tactics rather than taxonomies and nowhere is that need greater than in the areas of meaning and life purpose. The people we are serving do not need and can't make any use of abstract philosophical discussions. Instead, they need tactics and specifics.

For instance, a humane helper might suggest that her client learn "the habit of quick meaning repair." Every day we're bombarded by small and sometimes large threats to our experience of life as meaningful. Maybe you're a writer and get a particularly painful rejection. Suddenly writing and even life itself may seem that much less meaningful. Or maybe you've invested meaning in your home business. Just as you're about to launch your product, you notice that someone has beaten you to the marketplace. You're likely to experience that bit of bad luck as a blow to your sense of the meaningfulness of life. Here's where the habit of quick meaning repair would come in supremely handy.

First, you would recognize that something important has happened. You would admit that an existential blow has occurred. Second, you would feel the feeling. Emotional health isn't helped by denial. Third, you would remind yourself that meaning, because it is a psychological experience, is a wellspring and a renewable resource and that you can make new meaning as soon as the pain subsides. Fourth, you would actually make new meaning by taking appropriate action. You would send out your novel again or you would actively market your product despite the unexpected competition.

When a meaning crisis occurs, we become emotionally unwell, usually calling the experience "depression." Rarely do we recognize that a negative meaning event has occurred and that, in order to feel better, we must take action by making new meaning. It is therefore highly useful to acquire the above four-step habit: understand what's happened, feel the feeling, pledge to make new meaning, and make some new meaning. All of this a humane helper might teach. There would be no need to invoke the ghosts of Hegel, Kierkegaard, Sartre, Camus, or other existential writers. By creating simple, sensible, effective tactics like "the habit of quick meaning repair," a humane helper could prove of great help even in the elusive territories of meaning and life purpose.

Another simple tactic that a humane helper might teach is to suggest that her client create a menu of meaning opportunities (having first explained what that phrase means); envision a day that includes some meaning opportunities along with life's other tasks, chores, and responsibilities; and then try to live such a day. As simple as this tactic is, it represents valuable, even life-changing work that people rarely attempt. Here is the report of a participant in one of my life purpose boot-camp classes after spending a week with the above assignment.[2]

> I have considered myself for quite some time to be a "meaning" sort of person, that is, on a quest to find and live a meaningful life. But in thinking about meaning opportunities I began to realize that I had not deeply or practically considered what "meaning" is or what it entails to live a meaningful life. My past efforts have very much been focused on a kind of heavy-handed "making meaning," often with inconsistent, disappointing, or confusing results. Shifting to "an opportunity mindset" was huge for me. There was a wonderful feeling of relief. Not every attempt to "find meaning" has to succeed!

We have opportunities, and some may pan out, and others may not; and eliminating the sense of failure if meaning isn't experienced takes the pressure off from the get go.

As I say, realizing that the menu includes opportunities as opposed to guarantees took the pressure off. I was then much more able to approach this exercise in a fun, curious and expansive way. When I first sat down, I started with general categories (spending time with family, watching a beautiful sunset, etc.). But as I was going about my day, I became mindful in a much more specific, practical way of moments occurring that were meaning opportunities. I also knew that the exercise was rumbling around somewhere in the background of my brain. I'd be driving or doing something else other than this exercise and all of a sudden, a specific experience would pop into my brain and shout, "that was a meaning opportunity!" I loved this!

I also realized that much of my day is spent in non-meaning opportunity things. I particularly struggle with shifting from the way of life I've lived until recently (a workaholic unfulfilled lawyer) to a new way of living a flourishing and meaningful life. At the bottom line, I hit the question of how do I make an income to support myself when the items on my meaning opportunities list seem mostly intangible (a heartfelt conversation with my son, belly rubs for my dog)? As I've struggled with this issue this week, one exciting alternative came to mind. I'm going to try to take my current period of unemployment as a super-large meaning opportunity to chart my next course and to pay real attention to the idea that we pick our own life purposes. By engaging with this simple exercise of "creating a menu of meaning opportunities" I feel like I am getting closer to the underneath of things.

It is easy enough to visualize a contemporary "meaningless" day of the sort that most of your clients are likely experiencing. You wake up, get on your treadmill of obligations, get into traffic, spend an hour getting to a job that does nothing for you except pay the rent, spend eight or more hours there, get back into traffic, arrive home, fret about dinner, handle some more obligations like bills and family crises, and try to find a program on television that will take your mind off the fact that you have not lived any of your life purposes or made any meaning on that day. The reality of this sort of day demoralizes people everywhere, and the specter of it haunts young people who want something different but have no idea what that different life might look like.

Given these realities, it is clear why so many people opt for denial, chase meaning substitutes, and never live their life purposes. Humane helpers must not be afraid to face these client realities. Yes, there may look to be few good answers, given a client's present circumstances. Yes, this may go far beyond "diagnosing and treating" made-up mental disorders. Yes, this may take a humane helper into territory that he is not trained to navigate and which he may not be navigating that well himself. But to ignore his client's meaning and life purpose needs is to not help enough. A humane helper will go right there and say, "We have some difficult things to look at, ready or not." Our humane helper may not be fully ready and the person sitting across from her may not be fully ready either, but the inquiry will nevertheless begin.

Clients may well have trouble bringing up these needs, challenges, and difficulties, since they are much more accustomed to thinking of their distress in terms of "depression" or "bipolar disorder" or "ADD" or "generalized anxiety" or "PTSD." This is the language that the culture and the dominant paradigm use and it is likely the language that your client will use too. Therefore, it will probably fall on your shoulders to wonder aloud in this territory and help your clients acquire new language, tactics, and strategies. You might begin to practice this "wondering aloud" with a helping buddy, in your dyadic work in your training program, or in some other way.

Humane helpers are obliged to come to a personal understanding of the value of discussing meaning and life purpose issues with clients or else they won't bring these matters up of their own accord or deal with them very well when clients bring them up. They are obliged to come around to valuing the importance of meaning and life purpose in human affairs and, having made that pivotal change in outlook, demand of themselves that they include life purpose, meaning, and value in their conversations with clients. Likewise, they must arrive at some concepts about meaning and life purpose that they themselves believe in and understand. If you yourself have no idea where meaning resides, how a conflict in values can be resolved, what it takes to make a strong life purpose decision and then stand behind that life purpose decision, how helpful can you be in helping others make meaning and live their life purposes? This is all part of a humane helper's self-work.

There is no reason why we can't begin to take a sophisticated view of the relationship between life purpose, meaning, and value, on the one hand, and distress relief, mental wellness, and physical wellness, on the other. In this sophisticated view, it will become better understood that human beings might want to exhaust themselves in the service of some life purpose and by so doing create distress and physical problems; yet at the same time, even as they create that distress and difficulty, they may be providing themselves with exactly what they need, psychologically speaking, and even be creating "genetic happiness," that deep happiness that comes from living our life purposes, experiencing meaning, and expressing our values.

In this sophisticated view, it will be understood that both can be true, that living as a value-based meaning maker can hurt, but that it can also help. We will begin to accept—even honor—the distress that arises because we have decided to fight for some cause close to our heart, struggle with some mind-breaking scientific problem, or paint the ceiling of our Sistine Chapel. We will then work to reduce that distress, insofar as that is possible, without calling the cause of that distress, our meaning-making efforts, into question. We will never say, "Don't make meaning—it is causing you too much distress." Rather we will say, "What can we do to reduce your experience of distress even as you pursue your meaning-making efforts?"

A lot of emotional and mental distress arises because an individual has never articulated his life purposes to himself, doesn't currently have any life purposes, doesn't know how to create meaningful experiences or answer his meaning questions, or is otherwise confused or bereft in the areas of life purpose and meaning. Humane helpers ought to be aware of this and should train themselves to work in this territory. What matters more to their clients than leading a meaningful, purposeful life? Humane helping takes this very human reality into account and takes seriously the pain that existential crises create.

POINTS FOR REFLECTION

1. Do you feel comfortable chatting about meaning and life purpose with clients? If not, what do you suppose is the source of that discomfort?

2. Do you see the value or virtue of chatting about meaning and life purpose with clients? If so, how might you introduce that conversation into your practice?

3. What are your own views about meaning? Do you believe that it is a singular, objective thing ("the meaning of life") that must be searched for and found or do you believe that it is a certain sort of subjective psychological experience that clients can cultivate?

4. What are your own views about life purpose? Do you believe that it is a singular, objective thing ("the purpose of life") or do you believe that individuals must make multiple subjective life purpose choices?

5. Describe in your own words how you might chat with clients about "meaning investments," "meaning opportunities," and "meaning repair."

NOTES

1 In private correspondence.
2 In private correspondence.

REFERENCE

Williams, P. (2012). "Brain Disease or Existential Crisis?" *Mad in America*. www. madinamerica.com/2012/08/op-ed-schizophreniapsychosis-brain-disease-or-existential-crisis/

11 Including Circumstances and Experiences

Let's say that I work in a factory, the factory is taken over by new ownership, and I'm told that I must triple my output, which is actually a physical impossibility. I try as hard as I can, I manage to double my output, and I am told that I will probably be fired for "not meeting expectations." I despair; I grow anxious; I stop sleeping well; I fight with my mate and yell at my children; and I arrive at the office of some designated helper—a clinical psychologist, my parish priest, a life coach, a Jungian analyst—looking for help. What will help me?

Will it help me to have my dreams interpreted? Will it help me to be repeatedly asked how I'm feeling? Will it help me to explore whether my thoughts are distorted and if it might help to substitute other thoughts? Will it help me to explore my childhood experiences? Will it help me to enumerate the ways that I feel distressed so that you can draw a symptom picture and provide me with a pseudo-medical-sounding label and a pill? Is any of that genuinely on point or helpful?

If we don't get to the heart of the matter, that my current reversal in circumstances is distressing me horribly, we will have missed the boat. It wouldn't matter how sympathetic, compassionate, kind, wise, or humane my helper was—except, of course, that I will appreciate all of that—we would still not be on track, not if it never came out that I am probably about to lose my job and that this prospect terrifies me; and that I am furious to the point of seriously considering revenge. That you are kind doesn't help me with any of that. Worse still is if you spend a bare fifteen minutes with me, act as if I am having some biological malfunction, call me clinically depressed, and write me a script for a chemical.

If you, my helper, are operating from the current paradigm and the pseudo-medical model, soon I will be unemployed, because I haven't been helped to deal with my current reality, and on an antidepressant, because my despair will get me a clinical depression label. Maybe, if I can afford them now that I'm unemployed, I'll also be taking chemicals for my anxiety, my insomnia, and my other "symptoms"; and my interactions with you will primarily be about dosages and compliance and side effects and drug cocktails and not about how my life has collapsed.

If you, my helper, are operating from the "expert talk about psychological issues" model—that is, if you are a psychotherapist of one sort or another—we will talk about many things, or perhaps I will talk and you will sit there and listen, and how we proceed will depend entirely on what you are accustomed to talking about: my dreams, my feelings, my coping skills, my distorted cognitions, my childhood experiences, my relationships, and so on. What we are unlikely to talk about, as it feels too mundane, too practical, not "psychological" enough, and even a violation of your mandate or your theoretical orientation, are my actual circumstances and how desperate they are making me feel.

How might a humane helper go about providing me with more help than this? First, I would certainly want to feel supported and heard by you. Without that solid ground, I wouldn't feel inclined to listen to you or "be there." Second, I wouldn't want my situation pathologized and I would prefer not to leave with a diagnosis and a prescription. Third, I would prefer not to have spent my time describing my childhood, my dreams, or my feelings. I would want my humane helper to say to me, "This is a very hard moment, isn't it?" and "Something's got to change, yes?" and especially, "Let's see what we can do about all this despair, anxiety, insomnia, and rage while at the same time focusing on dealing with this terrible employment thing."

I certainly wouldn't want you to administer an aptitude test or function as my career counselor. Nor would I want you to provide me with some abstract system for making a change, some "five steps to moving forward" plan or some "seven principles of authentic growth" exercise. Instead, I would love it if you asked me questions like, "Can you help me understand what's possible here?" and "Do you have any first ideas about how to improve your situation?" and "Given your ideas about what might be smart to try, what might get in the way of you actually making those changes?"

This last question is a strategically expansive question. It allows me, your client, to respond from any place I choose, from a so-to-speak practical place ("I need to keep making mortgage payments" or "The kind of work I do is vanishing"), if that's the sort of response that wants to percolate up. It allows me to respond from a so-to-speak psychological place ("I've never really felt equal to taking risks" or "My confidence is so low I don't think I can do anything"). Or it allows me to respond from a so-to-speak historical place ("As a kid, I once tried to express what I was feeling and got slapped" or "The last time I tried talking back to a boss I got fired instantly"), if a particular experience seems to me important to report.

This last response, that I was instantly fired the last time I tried talking back to a boss, is clearly an experience that matters to me, since I brought it up in response to your open, expansive question. Of all of the answers that I might have given you, this was the specific answer that percolated up. That likely signifies that my past experience of "being instantly fired" is one of my more important or meaningful experiences, certainly in this context. As such, mustn't it be worth our time to investigate it more fully? No matter where, as a helper, you had intended to go next (if you had any particular intention), doesn't it make sense to stay here with me and learn a bit more about that particular experience?

Therefore, you might proceed by saying, "Tell me about that." This gives me the chance to recall an experience that I am clearly holding as important (and maybe traumatic) and the opportunity to think through its current implications. I am probably going to fall silent for a while as I recall that time (if I respond instantly, am I really recalling it at all or just repeating some canned response that I've memorized to explain what happened back then?) and you will need to use your skill of sitting quietly and letting me think, rather than getting anxious and making me feel rushed. We will sit quietly there for a bit, I will think about that experience, and eventually I will respond.

As I think about that experience, both silently and out loud and with your help and your prompts, I may come to realize something important. For example, I may come to remember that after that firing I quickly landed another job, that new job much improved my life, and therefore I probably shouldn't be holding that "sudden firing" as a "traumatic experience" but rather log it in the column of "positive experiences." Wouldn't I find that interesting and encouraging? Might that not even change my whole attitude toward my current situation and give me the strength to make the change that we both know I need to make?

I might learn for myself, by talking it out with you, that without really being aware of it that past experience has caused me to freeze up in the present; and now, having aired that event, I may find it much easier to quit. This is one possible, natural and perhaps valuable outcome of you inviting me to recall that experience. At worst, we will have spent some time discussing something that I intuitively know must be relevant and I will appreciate your offering me the opportunity to do that recalling. I will have the sense that you "know what you're doing" and you will have gained a measure of my trust, which measure will allow you to venture in difficult areas more easily later. I will trust that you probably have good reasons for "going there," wherever you would like to lead me, because I have come to feel that you are both smart and on my side.

Let's say that it turns out that I can't leave my job, at least for now, either for practical reasons or for psychological reasons. It becomes clear to you, my humane helper, that I am "stuck" there; and likewise becomes clear to me. What help do I need from you now? I need you to help me cope, I need you to help me envision a good life that includes exactly these painful circumstances, and I need you to help me retain some hope for the future. That I can't change my circumstances doesn't mean that we can stop taking my circumstances into account. They are still real, pressing and even determinant of my emotional health and we have to figure out something to do to make my current situation better or at least bearable.

REFLECTING ON AN EXPERIENCE

If you've decided that giving clients homework between sessions is a useful idea, one sort of homework that you might give a client is the following. You might suggest to your client that she reflect on and write about a particular experience, maybe one that's come up in the current session or one that she's mentioned previously.

For example, a client of mine explained in session that it had recently occurred to her that the reason she had lost her self-confidence, a fact that was causing her great distress, had something to do with the way she'd handled the last day of her mother's life. I wondered if she thought that reflecting on that experience and writing about it might serve her. She thought that it might and she embraced that as her homework.

Her reflections proved very useful to her:[1]

Ever since my mom died two and a half years ago, I have felt very self-conscious. While I was caring for her, acting as her power of attorney and medical proxy, I had no trouble appraising situations and making fast, sure-footed decisions. This was true in all areas of my life. I felt confident in the work I did for my job. I confidently worked on writing novels. I had no trouble making decisions anywhere in life or understanding what I wanted, liked, disliked, or believed.

Now, I second-guess myself constantly. It is affecting my work. It has affected my writing. It irritates my husband. Even little things, like what should we have for dinner, have me wringing my hands. I know that I need to regain that confidence. But what robbed it? As I think about it, it's the irrational feeling that I could have and should have saved my mother's life, that there was something I could have done about her cancer, and that she didn't have to die on the day she died if only ... what? It's completely irrational; but from that day forward I've felt like a weakened version of myself.

I know that I did the best I could for my mother. I have proven myself to be a capable and thoughtful individual, in life and with regard to caring for my mother. I can't change the events of her last day. Even if I could, I don't believe I would change very much. I couldn't save her. She had cancer. Her heart and kidneys couldn't take any more drugs. I couldn't change that. No decisions I made would have changed that. How strange that I think that there was something else to do! What am I thinking?

Will this insight help me? I hope so! I know that I'm good at my job. I need to remember that I would not be doing this job if my boss didn't believe that I was the best person to be doing it. I need to trust myself again. I need to start writing again. I need to keep telling myself that I can do whatever I need to do and want to do and remind myself that others think I am capable and that I should believe them. I need to work on believing in myself. And I need to forgive myself for ... for what, for not preventing my mother from dying? Enough of that! Enough of that already.

Not every time a new client walks in will his or her current circumstances matter quite as much as in my example of a stressed-out, over-burdened factory worker. But very often they will. Circumstances really do matter. If, for example, a child has had his own room and suddenly must share it with a sibling and he begins to act out, it should be obvious that knowing about his changed circumstances is relevant, important information. Likewise, if his school lunch program shuts down for lack of funds, if now he is forced to skip lunch, and if "for some reason" he seems lethargic in the afternoon, surely knowing that he is no longer eating lunch would be information worth having.

This is all obvious; yet our current mental health system, with its twin focus on "mental disorders" and "psychological issues," casts a rather blind eye on a person's actual circumstances, whether that person is an adult or a child. Our humane helper will know better than to cast such a blind eye and will do an excellent job of inquiring about her client's circumstances. She will do this by asking simple questions like "What's been going on lately?" and "Has anything in your circumstances changed?" and "Paint me a picture of how you're living."

Her starting place is the presumption that circumstances matter and that she may well not hear about her client's relevant circumstances unless she asks about them. For one thing, clients are primed nowadays to presume that they will be hearing that they "have something" like a "bipolar disorder" and so may not be thinking that their circumstances matter or need to be reported. Because this is our current system, our humane helper knows that she must actively ask about her client's circumstances. Therefore, she might include this asking on her intake form, as part of her first-session investigating, at the beginning of every session, or in some other way. In whatever way she does it, she will remember to do it.

She will likewise inquire about her client's experiences. While she can't predict how a given person will be affected by a traumatic experience, by multiple traumatic experiences, by ongoing trauma, or really by any experience, positive or negative, a humane helper knows that experiences matter and that she wants to know about them and pay attention to them. Given that the average amount of time a psychiatrist spends with a new patient has shrunk to fifteen minutes, a humane helper has to wonder whether the dominant paradigm allows for experiences to be given their proper due—or any due. She reminds herself that in her helping practice she will not minimize their importance and she invites the person sitting across from her to describe and explain his lived experiences.

These experiences may have happened a long time ago, just last week, or any time in between. I was working with an Asian physician, a surgeon, who moonlighted as an actor and who had several nice credits on his acting résumé. Several months previously he'd fallen into a tailspin; ever since he'd been feeling sad, anxious, and confused. Now he was contemplating giving up acting. I asked the obvious question which, however, helpers often forget to ask: "Can you put your finger on anything that's happened recently that might account for this tailspin?"

He could. Just before the tailspin he'd landed a part on an episode of a popular television show, gone in to do the shoot, and royally messed up his lines several times in a row. No one admonished him but he knew that his performance had been anything but suave or professional. We both completely understood why he might feel terrible about such an unfortunate experience; but why so terrible? Why was he calling the very enterprise of acting into question because of one bad shoot and why had he sunk so low from that one mildly unfortunate experience?

We investigated this and learned something interesting. He had sunk so low by virtue of the power of analogy. When he wore his surgeon hat, no messes were permissible. There the consequences of mistakes were drastic. As a true professional, he couldn't countenance surgical mistakes and in the surgical arena he had set the bar at "perfectionism." But he had somehow set the bar there for his acting performances as well and was holding his mishap on set as disastrous as a mishap in the operating room.

It would have been very hard to understand his presenting distress without getting that recent botched experience on the table and without investigating its meaning. Once the power of that analogy became clear, he had no trouble putting his upset feelings to rest and actively resuming auditioning. To be sure, lingering issues remained. Performance anxiety persisted, as did some doubts about the value and appropriateness of acting. But this particular crisis had been handled—and without any need to label him or provide a chemical fix.

Given that life is one experience after another, producing a virtually limitless number of experiences in the course of a lifetime, which experiences does a humane helper focus on? She focuses on the ones that seem important to her and the ones that seem important to her client. Indeed, some of your client's experiences will rise to the level of life altering and life defining and naturally these deserve close attention. However, these may also be among the experiences that your client least wants to talk about.

Your client may be holding certain experiences as pivotal. At the same time, these may be the experiences about which he is most secretive. This truth, that the experiences we find most important are also the ones that we may feel most ashamed about or guilty about, is a powerful obstacle to self-knowledge, growth, and healing and likewise a powerful obstacle to a full exchange of information between client and helper. If I have a strong desire to keep certain experiences secret—a secret from others but also a secret from myself—that desire is likely to outweigh my other, real desire to improve my life or my desire to speak frankly with my helper.

For example, in working with a demoralized actress we kept coming back to a movie she'd made in Italy in which she'd been the lead. This spaghetti western had been successful, a feather in her cap, and a boon to her career. Yet every time we chatted about it I got the sense that something about the experience had saddened her and harmed her. Finally, she revealed her secret. When she arrived in Italy the first thing the director said to her was, "You're too fat for the role. But we've paid you, so we'll use you." This indictment—and what became her unshakeable belief that she really was "too fat for an actress"—still haunted her.

A humane helper has to sit quietly with this information and be "with it" before trying to "do" anything with it. Because this "being with" is hard to do, many helpers don't want to receive information of this sort. They would really prefer not to know about their client's seminal experiences because those experiences are often painful to hear about and because it is so difficult to know what to do with them or about them. Still, getting them on the table is vital, since these experiences are often our best clues about how cause and effect is operating in our client's life.

As a result of just one such experience a client may feel that he is not really a moral person—that his one act of cruelty outweighs all of his otherwise good behavior. He may feel that he is not really a capable person—that a particular failure has somehow canceled all his many successes. He may feel that he is not really a valuable person—that some painful experience of unworthiness or humiliation is legitimate grounds for self-loathing. Experiences matter and a single experience, however objectively small or slight, may matter profoundly. Nor do they have to be negative experiences to be important and prove pivotal. A bit of praise from a client's third-grade teacher may buoy a whole writing career. Both negative and positive experiences matter and a humane helper is interested in these and is careful not to rush past them or gloss them over.

It should of course go without saying that a person's current circumstances and pivotal experiences matter. However, we seem to understand that about ourselves better than we understand that about other people. Since we may be a bit blind to the importance of circumstance and experience in the lives of the people we have decided to help, we may have to actively practice reminding ourselves that we should regularly check in on both.

Do you really not want to know that your despairing client has failed the bar exam four times already and is facing a fifth try next month or that your anxious client has been in three significant car crashes and is starting a cross-country trip with her young children in two weeks? In the pseudo-medical model of helping none of this is relevant and in many versions of the expert talk model this is likewise considered irrelevant information. I hope that makes no sense to you and that, as a humane helper, it becomes second nature for you to inquire about your clients' current circumstances and important life experiences.

POINTS FOR REFLECTION

1. How much emphasis do you currently put on investigating a client's circumstances?

2. Do you think it would be wise to do more investigating in that area?

3. If you do, how might you integrate that increased investigating into your practice?

4. Do you currently ask your client which experiences he or she believes were pivotal?

5. What changes might you make to your practice, if any, so as to better understand your client's circumstances and experiences?

NOTE

1 In personal correspondence.

12 Eclecticism and Personality Trait Work

A significant impediment to humane helping is relying too heavily on your theoretical orientation.

The idea that you must do things in a certain way and view human beings in a certain way—that you are exclusively a chemically oriented psychiatrist, a cognitive-behavioral psychologist, a Freudian analyst, a gestalt psychologist, an Adlerian, a self-psychologist, a narrative therapist, a Rogerian, a Jungian, an existential therapist, a Bowenian family therapist, etc.—is by its nature limiting. If you decide to stick tightly to the dictates of your theoretical orientation and don't allow for other ways of thinking and other ways of operating, you are in effect saying, "My system has the only right picture of who you are and how you can be helped."

Either intuitively or quite consciously, most helpers understand this limitation on relying too heavily or single-mindedly on their theoretical orientation. They therefore prefer to think of themselves as "eclectic." This tends to mean in practice that they take from their theoretical orientation what they like and what they actually believe in and leave the rest behind; and, likewise, that they take what they like and believe in from other theoretical orientations and freely use those ideas and techniques. This is a wise practice, as it allows helpers to pick and choose what they believe works—and what they believe works most humanely.

For example, maybe you are "essentially" cognitive-behavioral in orientation but you use a bit of "chair work" from gestalt therapy, certain thoughts about "disidentifying" from psychosynthesis, and the idea that human beings begin whole and start to become undeveloped until a midlife crisis strikes, a Jungian idea. Most practitioners in the real world operate like this, lifting from here and there and then staying with what seems to work, irrespective of what their theoretical orientation suggests or demands that they do. They opt for experience over theory and pragmatism over allegiance.

Indeed, where did the idea of needing a "theoretical orientation" come from? Helpers tend to acquire a theoretical orientation because an orientation feels particularly congenial to them (for example, the religious will be drawn more to Jung and the atheistic more to Freud), because their school focused on one and specialized in it, and/or because their licensing procedures demand that they "get grounded" in some theoretical orientation. But the idea is actually odd. Imagine a surgeon having a "theoretical orientation," as opposed to doing what's surgically sound. The very idea is suspect and resembles religious divisions more than science.

As a humane helper, your tasks are to think through to what extent you want to be a "strict" adherent of some theoretical orientation, to make sense of what you want "eclectic" to mean for you, to decide who you "essentially" want to be (for example, "I want to be as helpful as I can be" as opposed to "I'm a Freudian analyst"), and to pick those tactics, strategies, and ideas that you want to include from the countless theoretical orientations and ways of helping that are out there.

Of course, if one way of helping were objectively the best and the most helpful, then a humane helper ought to follow that specific course. But countless outcome studies on the effectiveness of psychotherapy have concluded that a client's report of a successful outcome is very little related to the theoretical orientation of the helper and quite robustly related to the helper's warmth and humanness. Three specific factors seem to account for the success of psychotherapy, when it's successful: the warmth and humanness of the helper, the willingness of the client to engage, and the very set-up, which allows a sufferer to unburden himself, think about his situation in a quiet room, and co-create solutions with someone who is listening carefully. The helper's theoretical orientation looks to count for very little in this picture.

What might this mean for you? Say that you are a chemically oriented psychiatrist who harbors some doubts about utilizing the DSM and some doubts about prescribing chemicals for what you suspect are problems in living and not pseudo-medical conditions. But your doubts do not lead you all the way to dropping the dominant paradigm as your theoretical orientation and your way of working. What might you add to humanize your practice, make it more eclectic, and better serve the people you see? Some psychiatrists add mindfulness training, spiritual investigating, trauma work, cognitive-behavioral work, ideas and practices from depth psychology, and so on. If you were a psychiatrist in this position, what do you suppose your particular eclectic mix might look like?

Or say that you're a cognitive-behavioral psychologist who wonders if your tactics and strategies around maladaptive self-talk scratch the surface sufficiently and help enough with intractable issues like long-standing trauma, a seriously pessimistic worldview, or high anxiety. If you have that sort of doubt or wonder, you might add depth work to your cognitive-behavioral work and acquire ways of helping your clients heal from trauma, rejigger their views with regard to meaning and life purpose, and reduce their experience of anxiety, say by learning some discharge techniques, relaxation techniques, or disidentification techniques. Even if you are a cognitive-behavioral psychologist, you are not obliged to always focus on a client's self-talk and behaviors. You can create and utilize an eclectic mix of helping strategies that allow you to go deeper than that.

Personally, I like to include "personality trait work" as a part of my eclectic mix. For me, this is a convenient way to think about, talk about, and focus on what I consider to be useful work with clients. As you may remember from your "theories of personality" class, if you happened to take one, personality trait theory (as championed by Gordon Allport and his cardinal traits, central traits, and secondary traits, by Raymond Cattell and his sixteen personality factors, by Hans Eysenck and his three dimensions of personality, and by others), was one of those fifteen or twenty theories of personalities that you glanced at briefly during that class.

I find the idea of "personality traits" metaphorically interesting and practically useful; without, of course, considering that personality trait theory resembles real theory. Theories of personality aren't genuine scientific theories. Rather they are collections of observations, opinions, suppositions, metaphors, and speculations. Indeed, calling them "theories of personality" is yet another place where psychology overreaches and uses loose language to impress itself, impress others, and act as if it knows more than it knows. No "theory of personality" has ever been subjected to the scrutiny of the scientific method, with its "high bar" demand of falsifiability: that is, that if experimental evidence contradicts your theory, your theory must change to accommodate that evidence rather than ignoring it or minimizing its importance.

No theory of personality has ever come close to meeting the rigors of science, not Freudian theory, Jungian theory, Adlerian theory, or any other so-called theory of personality. However much a so-called theory of personality may prove interesting, sometimes insightful, and valuable as metaphor, it nevertheless falls far short of deserving to be called a theory. It may, though, contain elements that are useful to you as a humane helper, elements that you can lift from that system and whose metaphoric power can help your clients. In that regard, I like personality trait theory.

One particular metaphoric view of personality is that we are collections of personality traits and that we as individuals—and as helpers—can isolate those traits, "work on them," and by doing that work reduce our distress and improve our personality. In the creativity literature alone more than seventy-five such traits have been identified as "making up" and valuable to a creative person, traits like concentration, confidence, curiosity, and cognitive flexibility. I find this metaphoric view useful and it helps me frame my work with clients, allowing me to say, for example, "Do you think it might make sense to work on your confidence?" or "It sounds like you're saying that you'd like to work on your concentration?"

Almost anything that we can say about a human being can be construed as an aspect of personality and a "personality trait." This is very useful for a humane helper. For example, you and your client can come to the conclusion that working on a particular personality trait or certain personality traits is a sensible part of your game plan; you can refine this idea by adding that it isn't always "more" of a given trait that's wanted, that sometimes it's "less" of a given trait that's desirable; and refine this idea further by arriving at an understanding of how traits interconnect. Indeed, one of your client's stated goals might be to "get all of my traits in right alignment so that I'm the person I'd like to be."

Isolating a trait and working on it can prove a rewarding experience for clients. A client might focus on becoming a better risk-taker, for example, by paying attention to that trait for a period of time and inventing exercises and tasks that help her take new risks. She could decide to tackle a project or a change in her circumstances—a novel, say, or a career change—whose bigness frightens her and which, in fact, she might never have been equal to contemplating except in the context of "working on risk-taking."

As a rule, clients will tend to manifest "too little" of a given trait and will therefore decide to manifest "more" of the trait or the traits they single out to work on. Your client might want to manifest more courage, more discipline, more imagination, more passion, and so on. On the other hand, a given client may want and need to manifest "less" of a certain trait: less skepticism, for instance, if her skepticism has slid into nihilism. There is certainly no rule that every client needs "more" of any particular trait; rather, each client needs the "right amount" of each trait and the "right integration" of all traits.

It is also possible that you will not actually name these personality traits out loud as you work with clients but rather keep them in your own mind as guidance. For example, your client may seem to rely too heavily on authority—on you, on a book she's reading, or on some religious, social, or cultural figure—and this may suggest to you that she is "insufficiently self-directing." Instead of saying anything to her about self-direction as a personality trait or about the harmfulness of insufficient self-direction, you might work "silently" on this issue by, for example, engaging in an in-session role-play where she is "the director" and you are "waiting to receive her directions."

Consider the "personality trait" of confidence, one that I'm obliged to work on all the time with my creative and performing artist clients. Most people tend to recognize that they do not feel as confident as they would like to feel. However, this recognition is often obscured by the fact that they may feel quite confident about some aspects of their life, at least fairly confident about some other aspects, and only unconfident in certain specific areas, say in situations like dating, speaking in front of an audience, or when they try to create.

They may work a day job where they supervise a dozen people or handle a budget of millions of dollars and feel confident about their ability to manage employees, get projects done on time, handle the never-ending interpersonal and practical problems that arise in the typical workplace, and so on. Therefore, when it comes time to create and they can't, they are not likely to identify "lack of confidence" as the issue, since, for most of their day, they have been acting quite confidently (or at least managing to look confident). Therefore, it may be our humane helper's task to wonder aloud about "confidence as an issue," since her client may not know to bring it up.

If you were wanting to add personality trait work to your eclectic mix, you could introduce the idea of "working on confidence" by saying something like the following:

> Mary, you indicate that you're having trouble getting your novel started and you seem to feel that the problem is your lack of a good idea for a novel. I wonder if the problem might be something else? Maybe you don't really feel confident about starting a novel at this time? Many people are less confident about launching a big creative project than they realize, so I find that taking a look at confidence is generally a good idea. What do you think?

If your client disagrees, you pursue a different avenue. But if she agrees, then you and she can co-create some tasks designed to "increase her confidence." You can work in this simple, useful way with any personality trait that you deem important. What personality traits might you decide to work on with clients? The list is virtually limitless. Here are a few, to give you a sense of the vastness of the territory: self-trust, openness to experience, optimism, empathy, discipline, assertiveness, concentration, courage, passion, playfulness, persistence, and so on. Virtually anything that you can say about a human being can be reframed and functionally treated as a personality trait.

One feature of personality that particularly interests me is "energy." It is not at all clear what energy, passion, vitality, drive, desire, or the life force are; or what distinctions we would want to make among these related but quite different concepts. But is there any "personality trait" that is more important than a client's "energy level"? How can a client manage to reduce her distress, make any necessary changes, or meet her goals if she is deficient in energy or somehow blocked with regard to energy? Indeed, doesn't her energy level affect the session itself? What "personality trait" could be more important to work on?

The question is not how you might go about defining "energy" or even how you might go about understanding it: this is no academic exercise. No definitions are really possible and no investigations are necessary. There is a whole Freudian literature just on "libidinal energy" and the "fixation" of that energy, a literature that treats energy as an amount and that speculates on the ways that that amount can be captured, arrested, or reduced as a result of unresolved intrapsychic conflicts. Another literature concerns itself with mania, a state that must have something to do with "energy"; a third literature deals with obsessiveness, which likewise must somehow be related to "energy"; and so on. We can't hope to get to the bottom of the mysteries of energy and life force and we don't need to. Rather, we simply chat about them with clients, employing their metaphoric resonance, and see if thinking about "energy" or "the life force" opens the door to useful insights for a given client.

What might this work sound like in actual practice? A humane helper might present the idea of "teasing apart energy and anxiety," with an eye toward having her client eliminate those "energetic activities" that are rooted in anxiety (like compulsive shopping or compulsive sex) and attaining some state like "calm wildness" or "measured passion." Just arriving at a metaphor like "calm wildness," which captures something of the paradoxical, complicated nature of an energetic balance that might prove useful to a client, is often therapeutic in its own right. Part of the task of helping a client effectively make meaning, heal from trauma, and reduce distress is arriving at metaphors like "calm wildness" that are rich in meaning.

A humane helper's client might, for example, feel more energetic if he conformed less. Our helper might provide a metaphor like "learned tameness" and, in cooperation with her client, dream up and maybe rehearse some conformity-busting homework. Or she might ask a question like, "What small, wild, energizing thing would you like to do this week?" Likewise, she might investigate whether her client is holding any social, cultural, or familial injunctions against displaying passion, which might prove to be yet another way of getting at his "deadness" and his lack of energy. It should be clear just how much rich work you might do in this area.

Or consider the "personality trait" of persistence. When we observe a screenwriter continue to work on her screenplay draft after painful draft, when we see an actor still audition after countless rejections, when we watch a sculptor chisel down his figure until it crumbles, only to start all over again, we are witnessing heroic meaning-making in action and the persistence required of a creative person. Persistence is required to build and maintain a career, to build and maintain relationships, to successfully deal with an addiction and remain in recovery, and in virtually every other aspect of life.

Say that our humane helper is a creativity coach. Because defensiveness can look like persistence and persistence can look like defensiveness, a creativity coach can't know right off the bat if her client should be supported in her adamant, stubborn path or advised to stop, reflect, and change. Is seven years working on a novel a persistence to be praised or a defensiveness to be confronted? Is it heroic to still be taking acting classes at fifty, despite not landing a part in a decade, or a defense against admitting that a new creative path might be wiser? You will only learn as you work with a client, hear him speak about his path, gauge his reality-testing efforts and his honesty, and otherwise gain an understanding of his particular story what is going on—and how you want to make use of the idea of "persistence as a desirable personality trait."

More people will manifest insufficient persistence than will manifest a too-stubborn persistence. Most people are not persistent enough. Disappointed, harmed by criticism, rejection, failures, and often early trauma, daunted by a lack of success, conflicted about the ultimate value of their pursuits, and otherwise undermined in their pursuit of a meaningful life, most people do not fight tooth and nail for their dreams, they do not continue on no matter what, and they do not persist in the face of the long odds against them. This is the usual story.

In working with this majority, a humane helper might, for example, wonder aloud whether her client holds "persistence" as a taboo quality that represents an assertiveness, independence, or autonomy not permitted in her family of origin. She might suggest to her client that he choose something to be "really persistent" about, even to the point of "overdoing it." She might frame persistence as a certain sort of habit and suggest that her client works on becoming "routinely persistent" and "persistent on a daily basis." She might float the idea that her client's lack of persistence might really be an inability to concentrate; and inquire if he would like to work on blocking out distractions, changing his cognitive landscape, quieting his mind, and learning to concentrate. Or she might wonder, "What is meaningful enough to warrant real persistence?" If her client can't answer this question, it naturally follows that there are meaning and life purpose questions to address.

A common shadow side of this rather necessary heroic persistence is over-stubbornness. It is probably overly stubborn to try to resume a dance career after hip-replacement surgery and against medical advice, overly stubborn to write in a genre whose time has passed, overly stubborn to persist in advocating for a flat earth or against continental drift. Stubborn persistence of this sort may be more a defense against the truth or a display of thoughtless ego than useful persistence. To work on this shadow side of persistence, a humane helper might ask a question like, "What do you think too much persistence looks like?" or "Do you think that sometimes too much persistence can be a problem?" and see how her client responds. Getting such questions on the table can in and of itself prove valuable work.

To repeat: you can treat personality as made up of building blocks or personality traits, each of which can profitably be worked on separately. Each personality trait can be conceptualized as a kind of amount and you and your client can think through if she is manifesting "too much" of it, "too little" of it, or "just the right amount." Each of these building blocks likewise come with a shadow side at both poles, the "too much" pole and the "too little" pole; and most clients will likely reside in the shadows at the "too little" pole, lacking genuine confidence, manifesting too little resolve, and so on.

You can profitably isolate traits to work on, if you choose to do so. A problem, issue, or place of distress can be framed in terms of personality trait work, for instance by wondering aloud if a client would like to work directly on "building confidence," "concentrating better," "growing more disciplined," and so on. Systems theory, the basis of much of family therapy, asserts that no matter where you intervene in a system, you affect the entire system. This is the logic behind not always needing the whole family in the room and still calling what you are doing "family therapy." In its own way, the same is true about personality trait work. Personality trait work, which at first glance looks atomistic, is in fact holistic: your "whole" client can be helped by focusing on any given personality trait.

Personality trait work is one sort of addition you might want to make to your eclectic mix. What will your particular eclectic repertoire of tactics and strategies look like? Part of a humane helper's eclectic work might involve helping her clients learn new skills and adopt new habits. Useful skills might include relationship skills, parenting skills, communication skills, business skills, personality trait skills of the sort I've just described, and so on; as well as useful habits that might include daily exercise, diet, recovery work, a daily creativity practice, and so on. The rubric for this focus is: "In order to get from here to where you would like to go, you will probably need to learn some new skills and acquire some new habits."

A humane helper might likewise focus on "change." She might help the person sitting across from her understand that any desired change involves actual change. If a client wants to feel less sad, less angry, less anxious, and less down on life and hopes to deal more effectively with the real world, certain efforts will be required. A way to get at this and help your client make these important changes is to focus not on the change per se—the divorce, say, or the career change—but on a quality or trait that, if it were more developed or if it were manifested more often, might help your client make that change more easily. This might be another reason to include personality trait work in your eclectic mix.

It may be the case that you are still quite wed to your theoretical orientation, in which case the idea of practicing eclectically may not sit well with you. If you follow the tenets of your theoretical orientation very closely, because you believe in them or perhaps because you like how it defines you professionally ("I'm a Freudian analyst"; "I'm a cognitive-behavioral psychologist"), you may not feel very sympathetic toward the idea of an eclectic approach. Still, I hope that you'll give the idea some thought. You must know that your theoretical orientation can't really amount to gospel, given that it isn't anything like proven theory. Since that's the case, do give the idea of eclecticism some thought.

What you gain by stepping outside the strictures and limits of your theoretical orientation, self-identifying as eclectic, and making use of additional ideas, tactics and strategies from "all over" that seem useful to you, may prove really valuable—and humane as well. Why humane? Because, by pulling from here and there what you believe works, you are honoring your commitment to helping and you are providing more help than if you slavishly adhered to some dogmatic system.

Maybe your client would really benefit from knowing about a certain therapeutic wilderness opportunity or some parenting skills class but maybe in your model of helping you are enjoined from offering recommendations of that sort because they "break the therapeutic frame." Does that proscription really make sense? There's so much that might help another person—why limit what you offer to one theoretical position? The main criterion a helper ought to use as she works with clients is, "Might this help?" and not "What does theory say I should do?" Many things might help: please do have permission to try them.

POINTS FOR REFLECTION

1. If you have a theoretical orientation, what do you see as its pluses and minuses?

2. To what extent to do you actually use your theoretical orientation in practice?

3. Explain in your own words the pluses and minuses of working eclectically.

4. Can you paint a picture of what your eclectic practice might look like?

5. What are your thoughts on including personality trait work in your practice?

13 Understanding the Psychiatric Survivor Recovery and Peer Support Movements

What helps a person in distress? Well, mustn't "what helps" be logically connected to the sort of the distress a person is experiencing and the source or sources of that distress? A brain injury, a year in isolation, hating your job, being sad by nature, and addictively surfing the Internet every night all produce difficulties but it makes no sense to suppose that "what helps" can be identical in each case. It wouldn't matter if the so-called diagnosis were the same in each case: that is, if all these folks happened to end up with a "clinical depression" diagnosis. The help we mean to offer logically ought to be related to what's actually going on and not to some label we affix.

In the mental health field, a distinction is typically made between those folks whose distress or difficulty is of one sort ("less severe") and those folks whose distress or difficulty is of another sort ("more severe"). That is, a distinction is commonly made between a "mild mental disorder" like an "adjustment disorder" (say, having a hard freshman year at college) and a "serious mental illness" like "schizophrenia" (say, having that same hard freshman year and also hearing voices).

The general assumption is that the former can be helped by measures like "expert talk" (psychotherapy), whether alone or in conjunction with so-called psychiatric medication, and can in a restricted sense "go away" (though the label never goes away); while the latter must be treated with chemicals, will always remain a problem, and predicts a lifetime of not only difficulty but likely impairment and disability.

What is usually connoted by the distinction between a "mental disorder" and a "serious mental illness" is that the former person can function in society better than the latter person, is still "rational" rather than "irrational," is better able to meet societal standards of behavior, isn't plagued by "peculiar" symptoms like auditory or visual hallucinations, is perhaps psychologically troubled rather than biologically impaired and, while troubled, is still in his or her "right mind."

As a helper, you may find yourself only rarely endeavoring to help people carrying a "serious mental illness" label—or, by contrast, you may find yourself working with them very often, maybe in a community of care setting or a custodial setting. Whether or not this is a population that you work with regularly, it's a good idea that you become aware of the psychiatric survivor recovery movement, the psychiatric peer support movement, and their points of view. Rather than believing that "you are schizophrenic, you will always be schizophrenic, you will always need to be on medication, and you shouldn't expect to have much of a life," psychiatric survivors and practitioners in the psychiatric survivor recovery movement believe "you may currently be hearing voices and having a very difficult time but, whether or not you continue to hear voices and continue to have to deal with major challenges, like coming back from a history of trauma, you can recover and live a good, high functioning, productive life."

Remember one of our most important headlines: we do not know. We absolutely do not know the source or meaning of phenomena like auditory and visual hallucinations and to affix a label like "schizophrenic" to a person with such experiences adds zero knowing to the equation. It makes a great deal of difference whether, as a helper, you smugly say "You are schizophrenic" or whether you say "We have no idea why you're experiencing what you're experiencing." The latter is the truth and allows for different approaches than just knee-jerk chemical dispensing. There may be times when chemicals with powerful effects are warranted and that may prove especially true when it comes to so-called "serious mental illness," but that a chemical might prove helpful is not proof that we know what is going on or that it is useful or justified in any particular instance.

Given this truth, that no one knows what a "serious mental illness" is or what best helps a person deal with it or recover from it, you can as legitimately point a sufferer in the direction of the psychiatric survivor recovery movement and the psychiatric peer support movement as in any other direction. You can humanely and compassionately say, "There are a lot of folks out there who predict a good life for you." Who are these folks and what are their positions? Let me introduce you to a few.

Dr. Eleanor Longden is a researcher, mental health activist and board member of Intervoice, currently based at The Psychosis Research Unit in Manchester, England. She lectures and publishes internationally on the importance of emphasizing person-centered, psychosocial approaches to complex mental health problems. She is a former TED speaker and the author of *Learning from the Voices in My Head*. Eleanor explained to me:

> When I was a teenager at university, I began hearing a single, neutral voice that calmly narrated everything I was doing in the third person: "she is going to a lecture," "she is leaving the building." Only the messages didn't stay passive for long. That day was the beginning of years of nightmarish voices, visions, and bizarre, terrifying delusions that drove me to self-harm in desperation, and led a psychiatrist to remark that I would have been better off with cancer because "it would be easier to cure than schizophrenia." Essentially, I was diagnosed, drugged, and discarded by a system that didn't know how to help me.
>
> A major turning point was encountering individuals from the Hearing Voices Network, who were willing to acknowledge and understand the experiences of trauma and abuse I'd endured as a child and young adult, and how these horrors from the past were still being enacted in the present. It was a long, torturous journey, but once I started to interpret my terror and despair in terms of what I'd survived, I could begin to recover: that my so-called symptoms of schizophrenia weren't random products of a chemical imbalance but rather meaningful messages from my mind about the unbearable things I'd gone through.
>
> I believe that recovery is a fundamental human right, and while there remains a great degree of pessimism about the capacity of people with "serious mental illness" to recover, the evidence shows that this is simply not true. A recovery approach, from my perspective, is holistic, person-centered, solution-focused, and an ongoing journey rather than a fixed goal or endpoint. I think it's also very important to broaden the focus from clinical recovery to incorporate the concept of personal recovery: factors like hope, identity, empowerment, subjective meaning and the ability to fulfill one's individual goals.

In my own personal journey, I spent many years stuck within the limitations of a coercive "cure" response, which emphasized factors like compliance, sedation, and silencing. In contrast, understanding, exploring, and engaging with the emotional meaning of my experiences was the recovery response. For many of us, an important part of personal recovery is the transformative process of making sense of your experience on your own terms, and using this knowledge to guide and inform genuine healing and growth.

Finally, it's also important that the concept of recovery is not used in a punitive or judgmental way. Complex factors like stigma, isolation, and hopelessness are major barriers to healing, and we need to recognize this and never blame someone for an inability to move forward in their recovery journey. There should be a profusion of compassion, support, and material and emotional resources for those that need them; yet there should also always be hope. To quote Pat Deegan, another well-known figure in this field: "It's important to meet people where they're at, but not leave them where they're at."

I think survivors must always be the authorities and authors of their own recovery process, but undoubtedly that journey becomes easier when you have allies to guide your way. There's a saying that it "takes a village to raise a child" and, in many ways, it takes a community to support a recovery story. For so many of us, the things that drive us mad, experiences of loss, trauma, discrimination, or injustice, take place on a silent, shameful, lonely stage. Recovery is the opposite: it's about reconnection and solidarity. This is why organizations like the Hearing Voices Network can be so enormously empowering, because although they maintain an unshakable belief in the power and resilience of the individual, they also provide a place for shared support and mutual understanding.

(Maisel, 2016a)

Or take Mark Ragins. Mark is a psychiatrist who has been at the MHALA Village since it opened in 1990. He's worked on their Full Service Partnership teams, their Homeless Assistance Program, their Transitional Age Youth Academy, and now on their Welcoming team and as their Medical Director. He's been heavily involved in the recovery movement for twenty-five years writing, speaking, training, consulting, and developing clinical and administrative tools to support their work. Mark explained to me:

> MHALA is a large local chapter of National Mental Health America. We operate a variety of programs centered around advocacy, public education, service delivery, innovation, workforce training, and community development. Our services are in two main clusters, one in Lancaster and one in Long Beach.
>
> The Village was established in 1990 initially as a demonstration project funded by the California state legislature. Some of the same legislators who had brought deinstitutionalization to California in the 1970s had serious misgivings about how community mental health had turned out. Too many people seemed to be falling between the cracks and ending up not getting the help they needed. They wanted us to demonstrate the best that community mental health could be.
>
> Administratively, we were integrated with capitated funding and quality of life outcome accountability. We soon found that the emerging recovery movement gave us the vision to integrate all those services into one welcoming, hopeful, vibrant program. An outside evaluator reported after three years that we had the best results across a range of quality of life outcomes of any program in the literature for people with a range of disabling mental illnesses. Visitors began coming to the Village from all over the world to be inspired and instructed. We became recognized leaders and proponents of the Recovery Model for people with mental illnesses.
>
> MHALA has moved from a "static" "services of indefinite duration" model to a "flow" model where people move along a continuum of recovery-based programs as they grow and recover. We now have a comprehensive recovery-based system of care in Long Beach. We designed the Milestones of Recovery (MORS) tool to track people's recovery and promote flow. We continue to innovate to improve our practice and push the boundaries of the recovery model while adapting to the ever-changing environment around us.
>
> We believe in the recovery model of care. We believe that recovery isn't something that can be done to someone. It is a process where people overcome the losses and destruction in their lives to rebuild themselves, their relationships, and their roles in the community. Recovery is a path best traveled alongside a helpful guide or mentor.

We use a model of four common stages of recovery (hope, empowerment, self-responsibility, and attaining meaningful roles) to help people live with dignity. The three major transformations in the recovery movement are:

1. Person-centered: Moving from centering our efforts on the treatment of illnesses and the reduction of symptoms to a holistic service of people and the rebuilding of lives. This is needed to engage people.

2. Client driven/collaboration: Moving from professional directed relationships emphasizing informed compliance with prescribed treatments to individualized relationships emphasizing empowerment and building people's self-responsibility. This is needed to motivate and build skills.

3. Strengths based/resilience: Building hope for recovery upon each person's strengths, motivations, and learning from suffering rather than upon the competence of professionals and medications to reduce or eliminate the burden of their illnesses. This is needed to build self-reliance and move on from depending on professionals.

(Maisel, 2016c)

A tenet of the psychiatric recovery movement is that psychiatric survivors can help and support one another, whether informally or in formal peer support organizations. Consider Jacqui Dillon. Jacqui is a respected speaker, writer and activist, and national Chair of the Hearing Voices Network in England. She is the co-editor of *Living with Voices: 50 Stories of Recovery, Demedicalising Misery: Psychiatry, Psychology and the Human Condition*, and the second edition of *Models of Madness: Psychological, Social and Biological Approaches to Psychosis*. She explained to me:

The Hearing Voices Network (HVN) in England is an influential, grassroots organization, which works to promote acceptance and understanding of hearing voices, seeing visions, and other unusual sensory experiences. HVN is a collaboration between experts by experience (voice-hearers and family members) who work in partnership with experts by profession (academics, clinicians and activists) to question, critique, and reframe traditional biomedical understandings of voice-hearing.

As the limits of a solely medical approach to hearing voices and other unusual perceptions becomes more widely known, and people become better informed about alternatives, there has been a growing acceptance by mainstream mental health providers of the approaches that we promote. Rather than being seen as a radical, fringe activity, HVN in England, which is probably the most well-established and well-developed network in the world, now has more than 180 groups operating in many conventional mental health settings, including child and adolescent mental health services, prisons, inpatient units, secure units as well as in community settings.

The position advocated by HVN—that hearing voices and other unusual sensory perceptions are common human experiences, for which there are many explanations—provides a much-needed antidote to the dominant medical discourse which deems these experiences as symptoms of serious mental illnesses, which need to be suppressed and eradicated with medication. Although some people find these approaches helpful, many do not. Finding a safe, confidential space to share your experiences with other people who are accepting of you and your voices, trying to understand the meaning of these experiences in order to make better peace with them, has been a transformative and healing experience for many.

Although the experience of hearing voices is solitary, complex, and varies from person to person, and some research suggests that hearing voices may be shaped by local culture, there are also themes that seem to be common for many voice hearers, across cultures. When I was working on *Living with Voices: 50 Stories of Recovery*, an anthology of testimonies from voice hearers from all over the world, what struck me was that even though each person's account was entirely unique, there were a number of key themes which emerged from all of the stories: that the voices were often a survival strategy, that the voices were deemed significant, decipherable, and intimately entwined to the hearer's life story, that voices sometimes used metaphorical language and that healing was not contingent on banishing the voices but about understanding their meaning, improving communication with the voices and consequently, having a more positive relationship with them.

The acceptance of a diversity of explanations for hearing voices, which is a central tenet of the HVM, has been crucial in developing the HVM internationally, without trying to export and impose Western ideas and assumptions about the mind or human experience. The HVM stance is one of respectful curiosity about the myriad ways people have of understanding voices, visions, sensory experiences, and altered states of consciousness. We seek to support people to make sense of their experiences, on their own terms. So, despite the well-established link between hearing voices and traumatic and adverse life experiences, the HVM explicitly accepts all explanations for hearing voices which may include an array of belief systems, including spiritual, religious, paranormal, technological, cultural, counter-cultural, philosophical, medical, and so on.

(Maisel, 2016b)

Last, here's Sascha Altman Dubrul. Sascha is a mental health activist, co-founder of The Icarus Project, an international community support network and media project working to redefine the culture of mental health, and the author of *Maps to the Other Side: The Adventures of a Bipolar Cartographer*. He explained to me:

One of the foundational aspects of Icarus has always been that it's a place both for people who take psychiatric drugs and those who don't, people who use diagnostic categories to define themselves and those who reject the labels—we believe strongly in harm reduction and self-determination. We have also always had a commitment to social justice, recognizing that so much of what gets called "mental illness" is interwoven with oppression: a system set up to divide us from one another and marginalize the people who aren't viewed as productive. From the beginning, we saw that if we were going to create a healthier safety net we would actually need to create a new language and culture that could reflect and hold the beauty and complexity of many people's diverse experiences.

Our society is so quick to pathologize difference and there is an institutional tendency to quell behavior that appears out of line and put it back in a labeled box in the service of the monoculture. That said, sensitive people like us are often our own worst enemies because we aren't taught the skills to recognize the signs of impending internal chaos and to know what to do. When you add growing social and economic oppression into the mix we find ourselves with a heavily medicated and/or incarcerated population of people who might otherwise be contributing to making our world a better and more beautiful place.

I think we need to begin by simply acknowledging how fundamentally flawed the current paradigm is—how little room it leaves for alternate views of health and wellness, how it privileges the knowledge of scientists and experts, and belittles the resources of local communities, families, and alternative health-care practitioners. We need to draw a clearer distinction between the usefulness of some modern psychiatric medications, and the reductionist biopsychiatric model that reduces our emotions and behavior to chemicals and neurotransmitters. We need to talk publicly about the relationship between unhealthy economic policies, the pharmaceutical industry, and our mental health. We need a vibrant social and political movement that has the wisdom and reverence for the human spirit and that understands the intertwined complexity of these things we call mental health, wellness, social justice, and global solidarity.

I think that whenever someone we care about is struggling with emotional or mental distress, it is often incredibly useful to seek the guidance of other people who have struggled with similar issues—learned from their experiences—and now have wisdom to share. I am a strong believer in the power of mentorship and peer support, the power of the wounded healer who has been through the fire of suffering to use their scars as guides to help others. I think one of the most important gifts we receive from our personal struggles is the ability to empathize and help others who have struggled like ourselves. This vision is missing from our current medical model, which puts so much of the power for healing into the hands of doctors and other experts. Anyone who I work with I see as a potential healer, a potential guide for others. I think having that vision reframes a key piece of what's wrong with the system.

(Maisel, 2016d)

In this chapter, I've focused on the psychiatric recovery movement and the psychiatric peer support movement. But the main point is more general. A humane helper can be of great help by knowing about, and alerting her clients to, those movements, organizations, and resources that provide peer support and frame the journey from "where you are" to "where you hope to be" as recovery.

These include well-established programs like Alcoholics Anonymous and Narcotics Anonymous and peer support programs without a recovery emphasis, for example peer counseling programs in the schools. A humane helper does not have to do everything herself and can't do everything herself. In fact, even imagining that to be possible is part of the problem we face with the current paradigm, which supposes that a person in distress is rather like a car and that a single mechanic can fix it. What a humane helper can do, in addition to trying to help her clients one-on-one, is point clients in the direction of other resources and other models, for instance but not limited to the psychiatric recovery movement and the psychiatric peer support movement, that might help them greatly. This pointing is an aspect of humane helping.

POINTS FOR REFLECTION

1. Do you have firsthand experience as a consumer of mental health services? What do you take away from those experiences that inform your practice?

2. In your view, to what extent should the experiences of "psychiatric survivors" inform your practice?

3. Describe in your own words what a "recovery model" signifies.

4. Which strategies, tactics, or tenets of the recovery movement might you like to incorporate in your practice?

5. Do you have the sense that learning more about the psychiatric recovery and peer support movement would or wouldn't prove valuable to you?

REFERENCES

Maisel, E. (2016a). "Eleanor Longden on Recovery-Oriented Approaches." *Psychology Today*. www.psychologytoday.com/blog/rethinking-mental-health/201602/eleanor-longden-recovery-oriented-approaches

Maisel, E. (2016b). "Jacqui Dillon on the Hearing Voices Network." *Psychology Today*. www.psychologytoday.com/blog/rethinking-mental-health/201605/jacqui-dillon-the-hearing-voices-network

Maisel, E. (2016c). "Mark Ragins on MHA Village." *Psychology Today*. www.psychologytoday.com/blog/rethinking-mental-health/201603/mark-ragins-mha-village

Maisel, E. (2016d). "Sascha DuBrul on Navigating Between Brilliance and Madness." *Psychology Today*. www.psychologytoday.com/blog/rethinking-mental-health/201604/sascha-dubrul-navigating-between-brilliance-and-madness

14 Humanely Helping Children

Most helpers do not work with children; but some do. When you work with a child of any age many special challenges arise having to do with who has the problem, the child or his or her family, to what extent it makes sense to see the child alone or whether only family therapy makes sense, the epidemic diagnosing of so-called mental disorders like ADHD and the amazing extent to which children nowadays are on prescribed chemicals, what amounts to the most age-appropriate sorts of helping, the extent to which you are there for the child or an agent of the parents, and so on.

In this chapter, let's look at the situation from a parent's point of view. The better you understand the challenges that parents face, the more humane and the more effective you can be as a children's helper. Shortly I'll describe fourteen questions whose answers are important to parents. Part of your task as a children's humane helper is alerting parents to these questions, as they rarely know to ask them or only have a vague appreciation of them; and providing some answers. You might even turn these fourteen questions into a checklist or handout of your own that you offer to parents and that you discuss with parents.

This may be an especially hard time to be a parent. In addition to all of the other stresses put on parents, from paying bills to dealing with a child's toothaches, earaches, and teenage years, now a parent has to deal with—and maybe protect herself from—the epidemic of "mental disorder" diagnosing (opponents of the paradigm would say labeling) that currently threatens millions of children and their parents. Indeed, you may find yourself in exactly this predicament and under this precise stress as a parent. What exactly is going on?

We have certainly come a long way in our compassionate treatment of children. We no longer look at children as a workforce; we see them as having rights and deserving not be abused; we believe that they have a right to be educated. Now, suddenly, in the course of just a handful of years, it looks as if we have taken a huge step backward. We are now rushing down the road of turning every feature of childhood into a "symptom of a mental disorder" and turning every child into a "mental patient."

Currently one in thirteen children are on so-called psychiatric medication. If you are a child and find yourself "in the system"—say in foster care—that number increases to one in four. And those numbers are increasing rapidly. What has happened? Primarily, certain ideas about "mental health" and "mental illness" have taken hold, promoted by special interest groups including psychiatrists and other mental health service providers and pharmaceutical companies, and that way of thinking became the dominant paradigm and continues as the dominant paradigm today.

Beginning in the 1950s, mental health professionals announced that if you displayed certain behaviors or had certain thoughts or feelings called "symptoms" you had a "mental illness." Despite the fact that they made this claim without any scientific justification whatsoever, this claim stuck. It continues to stick today—still without any scientific justification. The "symptom picture" model took hold—and now it looks to have grabbed us by the throat. Although this model makes no scientific or logical sense, it is our current standard of care and an extraordinarily profitable cash cow for pharmaceutical companies, researchers, mental health professionals, and other vested interests.

Because this is the dominant paradigm and because it is touted everywhere, including in the media and by parents themselves, wherever parents turn they hear about this little Bobby on ADHD medication or this little Sally on a cocktail of meds for her childhood depression. Bombarded with news about this supposed mental disorder epidemic and about the rising rates of diagnosis and chemical use, if their own child shows certain behaviors, thoughts, or feelings they are bound to suddenly fear that they have a "mental patient in the making." What could feel more terrible? Naturally feelings of helplessness, hopelessness, and failure are going to well up as a parent's very connection to her own child shifts from loving parent to frightened watchdog and prospective caretaker.

What might a parent who is worried about his or her child do instead of
or in addition to adopting the language and methods of the current mental
disorder paradigm? There are a great many things that he or she might try.
The following is just one sort of alternative, presented to give parents and
children's helpers a sense of an approach different from affixing a label
and proceeding with chemicals. Craig Wiener is a psychologist who wrote
the book *Parenting Your Child with ADHD: A No-Nonsense Guide for
Nurturing Self-Reliance and Cooperation*. Craig explained to me:

> I tell parents that a mental "illness" diagnosis means that their child
> is "doing" a set of atypical behaviors more often and with greater
> intensity than others do. Children do not "have" the category name.
> The name is a description of behavior and not an explanation of
> behavior, and there might be a variety of ways to account for why a
> child might qualify for the criteria of a mental health disorder. Instead
> of understanding their child's difficulties as a "chemical imbalance,"
> which is what most traditional interventions presume, the parent
> might understand their child's behavior as their child's way to cope.
>
> First, parents might observe and identify possible ways that day-
> to-day functioning reinforces the child's problematic behavior.
> Parents might then alter the sequence of events that are unwittingly
> perpetuating the unwanted patterns of behavior. Second, parents
> might use less coercion and less reliance on external cues or directives
> when helping the child meet socio-cultural expectations; this helps
> to develop autonomy and independence. Third, parents might
> incorporate the child's viewpoint as regularly as possible; this
> approach fosters amicable ways to resolve problems related to their
> child's integration with others. Fourth, parents can set firmer limits
> on the extent to which they will accommodate their child's behaviors
> during times of troublesome responding, and thus require the child
> to meet them halfway. Fifth, parents can role model the behaviors
> they want their child to imitate.
>
> (Maisel, 2016)

We might call the changes that Wiener suggests "more effective parenting skills" or "upgrading family dynamics." These changes might or
might not prove sufficient. By what if they did? What if, as a parent,
patiently working with your child, making changes in your family life,

and searching out services and resources like mentoring programs or peer counseling services improved the situation and spared your child a life-long label and powerful chemicals, chemicals whose negative long-term effects we are just beginning to understand? Wouldn't that prove a blessing?

Currently parents are bombarded by the mainstream view, fueled by pharmaceutical companies, academic researchers, mental health professionals, professional organizations, a naïve or indifferent media, and their own friends and family members, that "mental disorders" exist in the same way that "physical disorders" exist; and that if their child is afflicted with one of these "mental disorders," the only real help available are chemicals and perhaps also so-called expert talk called psychotherapy. However, these are not the only ways to look at the matter. Advocates of a critical psychology and a critical psychiatry approach suggest that there are other ways to conceptualize what's going on and other helpful approaches to take.

Certainly, chemicals may have their place in life—we are, after all, organisms that react to chemicals and sometimes a chemical fix may make sense. Practitioners in the critical psychiatry and critical psychology camps are divided on this issue: some see no place whatsoever for chemicals and others see a limited place for chemicals. What we all agree on, however, is that the current paradigm is pseudoscience and not science and that it is not the only approach to take when a child is experiencing difficulties or when a child's behaviors are causing him or her difficulties. There is much more to the picture than a label and a pill.

Each parent and each child who come into contact with the mental health system will have a different experience. Some parents may be happy that their "disruptive" child now has a diagnosis—that they now "know what's going on"—and may likewise be happy that "doctors are doing something for our child." They may swear by the chemicals that their child is given, happy for the short-term ameliorating effects and not overly concerned about any lasting side effects or about opening any pathways to addiction.

Other parents may have serious doubts about the legitimacy of the diagnosis their child receives, battle it a little, but finally "fall into line" when everyone, from school principal to teacher to learning specialist to general practitioner to psychiatrist, pushes for it. Some will find a wonderful family therapist who really helps; others may find a child psychologist or child psychiatrist who is excellent at helping; others may travel from practitioner to practitioner and remain essentially unsatisfied. Some will experience disastrous results, either because their child isn't really helped or because their child is made worse by the chemicals he or she receives. No single outcome or single story captures this very wide range of experiences.

However, this is definitely a "buyer beware" situation for parents. Proponents of the current paradigm believe that diagnosing via symptom pictures makes sense (as opposed to diagnosing via causes, as is done in medicine), that the book that describes these so-called mental disorders, the DSM, is a valid document, that defining a "mental disorder" is the same thing as proving that a "mental disorder" actually exists (of course the anxiety, despair, and other thoughts, feelings, and behaviors indubitably exist), that the chemicals with powerful effects prescribed as treatments for these so-called mental disorders are genuine medications (which of course they can't be if no medical illness is present) and other related, hotly disputed beliefs. I would ask parents and helpers to maintain a skeptical attitude, get informed, and see what they think.

If you are a humane helper who works with children, the following is a fourteen-point checklist for parents that you might actually use in your work with parents and their children and that, whether you use it or not, will alert you to the issues that you ought to be addressing. It speaks directly to parents, is framed from the parents' point of view, and might be used as is.

FOURTEEN-POINT CHECKLIST FOR PARENTS

If your child is experiencing difficulties or causing difficulties, here are a few questions to ask yourself, your child, the people in your circle, and, once they enter the picture, mental health service providers. These aren't the only questions you might consider—I hope you'll add your own questions to this list. But these are some important questions worth pondering:

1. *Is there a problem?*
   Let's say that your child is exhibiting some sort of behavior or having certain thoughts or feelings. First of all, is it a problem?

Is it a problem that your child waits two months longer to speak than did Jane across the street? Why is that a problem as opposed to a natural difference? Is it a problem that he enthusiastically signs up for violin lessons and then wants to stop them after two weeks? Why is that a problem as opposed to a change of heart? Is it a problem that he doesn't want to sit at the dinner table where you and your mate are fighting? Why is that a problem as opposed to good common sense? You can label any of these a problem—a developmental delay, a lack of discipline, a refusal to obey—but where is the love, charity, or logic in that?

2. *Has my child always been like this?*
   If your child has always been shy, why is it suddenly surprising that he or she is still shy now? If your child has always been bursting with energy and bouncing off the walls, why is it suddenly surprising that he or she is still full of energy and still bouncing off the walls? If your child has always been the quiet, brooding one, why is it suddenly surprising that he or she is still quiet and brooding? These may be features of your child's natural endowment or original personality or these may be features of his or her personality acquired so early on that they have pretty much always been there. Either way, there is no reason to treat your child's unique ways of being as suddenly surprising. His or her ways of being may create difficulties and those difficulties certainly must be addressed; but that isn't to say that your child suddenly "came down" with shyness, restlessness or brooding tendencies or that those qualities or behaviors are somehow markers of a "mental disorder."

3. *Have there been any big (or small) changes recently?*
   If a child's circumstances change, he or she is likely to react to those changes. Is your child in a new school? Doing new, harder schoolwork? Dealing with your separation or divorce? Living in a new town? Dealing with a new sibling? Did he or she move from a single room to a shared room? Have there been any

changes in diet or exercise? Maybe more junk food intake than usual or less exercise during a long winter? Changes in circumstances really do matter and you should think through if there have been any changes in your child's circumstances or your family's circumstances that may be contributing to or causing your child's current distress or difficulties.

4. *Is your child under stress?*
You might not think that your child having a prominent part in the school play might prove a source of serious stress for him or her, but it might. The same might hold true for an upcoming piano recital, spelling bee, or other public event or competition. Is your child taking a harder math class than last year or a history or language class that requires massive memorization? Challenges of this sort and many of the other challenges of childhood and the school years produce stress and that stress is likely to play itself out as distress and difficulty. Consider the link between stress and distress in your child's life.

5. *Has your child been abused or traumatized?*
Trauma and abuse produce distress. If your child comes home from summer camp and seems not to be his or her usual self, wouldn't it make sense to check in with your child to see if something abusive or traumatic occurred at camp? Has there been a death in the family, the death of one of your child's friends, or the death of a pet? Is your family life so chaotic as to rise to level of the traumatic? Has someone like a difficult aging parent recently moved into your home? Looking at matters from your child's perspective, might there be issues of abuse or trauma that he or she is trying to deal with (and maybe keeping secret about)?

6. *Who has the problem?*
If your mate belittles your child and your child grows sad and withdrawn, your child certainly has a problem. But isn't your mate the real problem? If you are highly anxious and vigilant and your child becomes highly anxious and vigilant, your child

certainly has a problem. But what's your part in the equation? If yours is a rigid and dogmatic household and your child rebels against your house rules, your child certainly has a problem. But isn't the family rigidity its own sort of problem? The question isn't about assigning blame or making anyone feel guilty. Rather it's a matter of appraising the situation honestly so that genuine answers can be found.

7. *What does your child say?*
   Have you asked your child what's going on? Asking is very different from accusing or interrogating. Have you had a quiet, compassionate, heart-to-heart conversation with your child in which you express your worry, announce your love, listen to your child's concerns, and collaborate with him or her on creating some strategies and tactics that might help your child deal with the problems that he or she is experiencing? Are you in the habit of checking in with your child to understand what he or she is thinking and feeling? If you haven't gotten into that habit, wouldn't that be a great habit to cultivate?

8. *What do other people say?*
   Have you checked in with the people in your circle: your mate, your other children, your parents, and anyone else who knows your child well? What are their thoughts about what's going on? They may have nothing useful or productive to offer or they may have some very important insights into what's happening. Ask the people who know your child well what they think. Make a special effort to check in with those people who seem the most levelheaded and whose opinions you respect the most.

9. *Do you feel kindly toward your child?*
   Human beings do not automatically love other human beings. Nor is love a stable, impregnable sort of thing. You may have lost patience with your child, feel oppressed by him or her, or in some other way have lost that loving feeling. Do you soften in his or her presence and want to hug your child or do you harden in his or her presence and do some scolding? What

child wouldn't grow sadder or angrier if he or she felt that what he or she got from a parent wasn't love but criticism or even revulsion? Think whether a softening and a more loving attitude might amount to great medicine.

10. *Are you quick to accept labels for yourself?*
How do you describe your own difficulties to yourself and to others? Do you say things like, "Oh, I have ADD and Bobby does too," "Depression runs in our family," or "We can't seem to get Sally's anxiety meds right—but I have the same problem myself"? If this is the way you speak and the way you conceptualize your difficulties and the difficulties of others, I would suggest that you educate yourself about alternate visions that reject the idea that because you have a certain experience, say of anxiety, you have a "mental disorder" and must take "medication" for that so-called mental disorder. I would ask you to be a little less quick to accept such labels for yourself or for your children and to engage in some "due diligence" research in this area.

11. *Has your child had a full medical workup recently?*
What if your child's school difficulties have to do with poor eyesight or poor hearing? What if his or her lethargy, pain complaints, or sleeplessness are symptoms of a medical condition? Make sure that you rule out genuine organic and biological causes for the "symptoms" that your child is displaying before supposing that they are "symptoms" of a "mental disorder." Of course, the root causes of human behaviors are not so easily traced back to medical conditions even when such conditions exist; but as possibly frustrating as the experience may prove, make sure that a medical workup is part of your plan to help your child with his or her current distress or difficulties.

12. *What sort of help are you looking for?*
You may decide that you alone can't do enough to help your child reduce his or her experience of distress. Where should you turn for help? It amounts to a very different decision to take your child to a child psychologist whose specialty is talk and

who uses techniques like play therapy or to a psychiatrist who routinely "diagnoses mental disorders" and who then "prescribes medication." There are many types of helpers out there, from peer counselor to school counselor to mentor to dietician to family therapist to residential treatment specialist to clinical psychologist to psychiatrist, and each comes at human challenges from a different angle. Educate yourself as to what these different service providers actually provide and decide which sort of service makes the most sense to you.

13. *A question to ask a mental health service provider: what is the rationale for labeling my child with a mental disorder and prescribing chemicals?*

If a mental health professional would like to give your child a mental disorder label, for instance the label ADHD, inquire as to his or her rationale for doing so. Ask questions like, "By 'mental disorder' do you mean 'medical issue'? If you do not mean 'medical issue,' why do you want to prescribe medicine to my child? If you do mean 'medical issue,' please explain to me what the medical issue is and what the evidence for it is." There are many more questions you might want to ask so as to satisfy yourself that the idea of "diagnosing and treating mental disorders" makes sense to you.

14. *Is my child actually getting better?*

Say that your child is placed on so-called psychiatric medication and his or her situation worsens. You will then be faced with the following very difficult questions. Is your child's condition actually worsening and is the so-called medication proving ineffective (and therefore perhaps ought to be changed or increased, which is likely what your child's psychiatrist will recommend)? Or is it the case that the so-called medication is actually causing the worsening (there is ample evidence that this can happen)? If your child's situation doesn't improve you are caught in the predicament of trying to figure out what's going on with your child and also needing to appraise the effectiveness or dangerousness of the help being offered your child.

> The above fourteen questions are a sizeable number of questions and, if you tackle them, will involve some perhaps painful self-reflection and a lot of investigating. But endeavoring to answer them will help you better understand what's really going on with your child and what will genuinely help him or her deal with his or her distress or difficulties.

Working with children is a specialty with many intricacies. It may involve you in reporting duties and contact with social services, it may stretch you in ways that excite you and that also make you anxious, and it may prove your most rewarding work. So very many parents are looking for help for their child different from a label and chemicals. And so many children are dealing with profound challenges—loss of a parent, divorce, poverty, bullying at school, abuse at home, or some other (or multiple other) "adverse childhood experiences"—and need that quintessential human support we've been discussing throughout this book.

They need the support of a real person who is willing to listen and who in a calm and practiced way can be with them just as they are, whether they are sad, silent, angry, fidgeting, sly, or otherwise themselves. They need the support of a person who is compassionate, kind, direct, brave, and savvy, who can hold the space and set appropriate boundaries, and who has educated herself about important resources that she herself can't provide, like peer counseling or mentoring. As younger and younger children find themselves forced into the mental health system, as a new wave of "prophylactic prescribing" is rearing its head ("Let's medicate kids who show no symptoms yet but who may show them one day"), and as more and more children find themselves on multiple chemicals, each with their own side effects, humane helpers who specialize in working with children are more needed than ever. Maybe this will become part of your practice—or your entire practice.

POINTS FOR REFLECTION

1. What are your thoughts on the current dominant paradigm of "diagnosing and treating mental disorders" as it pertains to children?

2. What are your thoughts on the current practice of prescribing "psychiatric medication" to children for their "mental disorders"?

3. If you work or were to work with children, would you consider it vital or not vital to work with the child's parents as well as the child?

4. How will you decide if the behaviors a child is displaying are "normal" or "abnormal"?

5. What do you see as some of the special challenges of working with children?

REFERENCE

Maisel, E. (2016). "Diagnoses as Descriptions of Behavior: An Interview with Craig Weiner." *Psychology Today*. www.psychologytoday.com/blog/rethinking-mental-health/201701/diagnoses-descriptions-behavior

15 Alternative Helping

Meaning Coaching

It is not the case that the only person who can help someone in distress is a certified or licensed mental health professional. First of all, mental health professionals are rather held hostage by the dictates, standard procedures, and paradigms of their license or certification, often meaning that they both feel obliged to "diagnose and treat mental disorders" and actually believe in that model, despite the lack of scientific evidence or logic supporting it.

Second, a sufferer's distress may really be better ameliorated by someone other than a certified or licensed mental health professional, for instance by a coach, workshop leader, instructor, mentor, peer counselor, AA sponsor, or a helper with some other self-designated specialty. Given that, for example, a licensed psychologist's training may have been primarily in the areas of testing and research and not in helping, whereas a mentor's whole focus may be on helping, who really is likely to be of more help?

If you are just beginning to think about how to be of help, you might go down the traditional path and become a licensed psychologist, psychiatrist, licensed family therapist, certified mental health counselor, and so on. Or you might go in some other direction entirely. Let's spend a little time looking at one specific, non-traditional way of helping: meaning coaching. A meaning coach works with individuals struggling with life purpose issues, endeavoring to identify their values and principles in order to make better life choices, and questioning whether their emotional problems like despair, anxiety, and addiction may be related to their meaning issues. They sometimes also work with institutions and businesses that want to clarify their mission and purpose.

Meaning coaching clients are likely to be experiencing the following sorts of challenges:

- They have the feeling that they are spending their days just going through the motions.

- They are unsure about where to invest their time and energy.

- They have the feeling that they are not really following their path or making use of their talents.

- They have trouble believing that their efforts matter.

- They spend a lot of their day feeling empty and listless.

- They're concerned that they need to make important changes but don't know how to make them.

- They have a career change or retirement looming.

- Meaning has always been something of an issue and challenge for them.

- They frequently second-guess their choices and keep switching from one path to another.

- They are frequently bored, anxious, or existentially blue.

Meaning coaches are first of all coaches. Coaching is the activity of one person helping another person. A batting coach helps batters improve their swing. A tennis coach helps tennis players learn court sense. An executive coach helps executives hone their people-management skills and their time-management skills. A creativity coach helps creative and performing artists break through blocks, create, and survive in the arts. A meaning coach helps clients identify their meaning challenges and works with them to create a more fulfilling life.

A good batting coach knows when to tamper with a batter's swing and when not to tamper with it. How does he know this? He knows this because he is thoughtful and observant about batting. He may never have been a great batter himself—maybe he couldn't get around fast enough on a major-league fastball—but he knows about batting because it interests him and because he is a student of the game. What is the game of which a meaning coach is a student? Life and its core issues, meaning and life purpose.

Imagine a client who presents the following issues. She does not feel fulfilled as a housewife and homemaker; she thinks she would like to write a mystery novel but doesn't know where to begin; she feels some hole or void that she usually calls depression but suspects is some kind of meaning crisis; she feels isolated and would like more friends; she also doesn't feel very sociable; she is worried about not contributing financially to the household; and more. This sounds like a lot and is a lot but it is exactly the sort of issue picture that a real-life client might present to a meaning coach or to any helper.

In this example, she has already "bought into" the idea that some meaning problem must be implicated here: remember, she has sought out a meaning coach. But she isn't sure what she ought to do and she isn't sure how a meaning coach might be able to help her. She is probably intrigued by the idea of receiving some meaning coaching but she also probably believes that her issues are as likely practical, psychological, and relational as existential. To put it simply, she is probably both hopeful and doubtful.

Say that you are a brand-new meaning coach. You may not have done much formal meaning coaching before; or much coaching at all, for that matter; or even entered into a "helping relationship" with that many people. At the same time, you probably believe that your life experiences count for a lot, that you have insights and a decent problem-solving skill set, and that you can probably be of help. You are likely exactly where your client is, doubtful and hopeful. However, it is on your shoulders to take the lead (even if you translate taking the lead as asking your client to set her own goals and name her own action steps) and so you must step right up to the plate.

You begin by listening; you start to conjure responses; you ask questions for clarification, if you do not understand; and at some point, you decide where you want to focus and how you want to reply. In essence, all coaches do the same thing: they provide the help a client is seeking by observing the client and responding to the client. Coaching is exactly that simple—and exactly that difficult. In this case, you might focus on any or all of the following, depending on how you want to work with this particular client and on what language she responds to the best:

- *You might focus on ranking issues.* This might sound like, "You've presented a lot of issues. Which one strikes you as the most important?

It might be smart to get these issues ordered in some way and then we can focus on the 'top' one to begin with."

- *You might focus on your client's intentions.* This might sound like, "I think that I'm getting that your intention is to break out of your role as homemaker and do something new and prospectively more meaningful. Have I got that right?"

- *You might focus on your client's value system.* This might sound like, "You've named quite a few issues. But I wonder if you can name some of your cherished values? Sometimes it's a good idea to get your values on the table and then choose your meaning investments based on what you value."

- *You might focus on your client's passions (or lack of passion).* This might sound like, "I hear that you want to write a mystery novel, but I'm curious if you're really passionate about writing one? Because mere interest usually can't sustain meaning—it often takes passion bordering on obsession. So, I wonder—do you feel passionate about your mystery novel? And if you don't, do you think we can get you 'more passionate'?"

- *You might focus on the idea of "opportunity."* This might sound like, "This is a golden opportunity to make some new meaning investments. You've named your mystery novel as one place that you'd like to make an investment. What sort of investment would you like to make in it and how would you like to make the most of this opportunity?"

- *You might focus on the idea of "meaning shifts."* This might sound like, "What would it be like to reduce your meaning investment in your housework and make a new meaning investment in your mystery novel? Do you think you might want to try making a meaning shift of that sort?"

All of the above approaches are secular and existential; that is, they are non-spiritual, non-religious, and non-denominational. However, what if your client announces that he is religious or spiritual? Then, in addition to any or all of the above approaches, each of which is congruent with a spiritual or religious belief system, you might investigate one or another of the following: you might ask your client how his spiritual beliefs inform his decisions about meaning; you might ask him to explain, as best he can, how he sees spirituality and meaning relating; you might ask him if he thinks that there is some spiritual plan that he must take into account as he thinks about meaning and, if there is one, what it is exactly; you might ask him what meaning he thinks he ought to make based on his religious beliefs or his understanding of God's plan for him; and/or you might ask him if there is anything in his belief system that conflicts with the idea of personal meaning-making.

What are your aims as a meaning coach? There are many ways to conceptualize your aims but one way is to suppose that you are helping clients in nine specific areas. You can present this to clients as "nine steps to personal fulfillment" or "nine ways to live with more purpose" or in any language you like. Millions of people feel listless, dispirited, and unfulfilled and so as to change their blue mood they play another computer game, take an antidepressant, keep very busy, and so on. But the listlessness and sadness typically remain. The following nine efforts can help change that picture:

1. *You decide to matter*
   The universe is not built to care about you. You must care about you. You must announce that you are opting to matter. You must announce that you are making the startling, eye-opening decision to take responsibility for your thoughts and your actions and live life instrumentally.

2. *You accept that you must make meaning*
   You finally let go of the demoralizing wish that meaning rains down on you from some golden universal shower and accept that the only meaning that exists is the meaning that you make. You announce once and for all that you are the final arbiter of meaning.

3. *You identify your life purposes*
   If you are going to actively make meaning in accordance with your life purposes, you had better know what your life purposes are, articulate them, and make sure that you really believe in them.

4. *You create a life purpose statement*
   You list your life purposes, rank order your life purposes, and do something with them that allows you to hold in a single phrase or

sentence a clear understanding of how you intend to live your life and how you mean to represent yourself.

5. *You hold the intention to fulfill your life purposes*
You need to keep your meaning-making efforts firmly in mind. You must be able to remember your life purposes even when you are tired, bothered, distracted, upset, and otherwise not in your best frame of mind. When life resumes its habitual busyness, you are obliged to still firmly hold your intentions and manifest them.

6. *You passionately act to fulfill your life purposes*
Every day you make some meaning in accordance with your life purposes. Maybe eight hours of your day are robbed by activities that do not align with your life purposes and that you must attend to for all the usual reasons. But some hours remain—and you must use them!

7. *You navigate the world and the facts of existence*
The world is not built to accommodate you. Your favorite bakery may close or war may break out—from the smallest to the largest, the facts of existence are exactly what they are. They include pain and pleasure, loyalty and betrayal, life and death. All this you must navigate, right up until the final moment.

8. *You create yourself in your own best image*
You have indubitable strengths and every manner of shadow. If you live in those shadows you will never quite respect yourself. Do better by manifesting your strengths and becoming the person you know you want to become. Surrender to the truth that you would prefer to be your best self.

9. *You live the life of a passionate meaning-maker*
You don't idly chat about meaning, brood about meaning, look for meaning, complain about meaning, buy a book about meaning, take a workshop on meaning: you make meaning. You live a life where, day in and day out, you make meaning. You make choices, decisions, and an effort. You wait on nothing: you live.

This is one sort of vision and one sort of program that a meaning coach might present to clients. Meaning coaches can also help their clients deal with their moods by reminding clients that they might want to focus more on their meaning needs and their meaning efforts rather than on the mood they happen to find themselves in.

We have gotten into the habit of taking the temperature of our mood far too often. Am I down? Am I very down? Am I down again? Am I down because I'm down? Hamlet pestered himself with the question "to be or not to be?" and rendered himself limp, passive, and indecisive. We pester ourselves with the question "Am I depressed or am I not depressed?" and fail to realize that this very checking in on our mood is a choice—and typically an unnecessary and unfortunate one.

What sort of answer would you expect if you checked in on your mood at a moment when you weren't actively making meaning? Naturally you would be "down," as you are checking in with yourself at precisely the wrong moment! You work for an hour on your novel and write a lovely scene. Do you check in on your mood as you're writing? No. You've been making meaning and feeling fine and see no reason to make note of your mood. An hour later, suddenly resistant to writing and uncertain about your novel's direction, you sit brooding on your sofa and then you decide to check in on your mood. Surprise, surprise! You notice that you're unhappy. Why check in at exactly that moment?

It is one of the universe's ironic little jokes that human beings check in with themselves about their mood at exactly the moment when it might be expected that their mood would be at its lowest. Rarely do we check in on our mood when we are having a good time or working hard on something engrossing. At those moments, it goes without saying how we are feeling—just fine—and so we don't bother to announce our good mood to ourselves. We wait until we aren't occupied and aren't actively making meaning to check in. How brilliant is that? A meaning coach can remind her clients about this common dynamic and help them focus on their meaning-making efforts and not on their moods.

Meaning coaches can also help their clients negotiate their days: that is, they can help their clients think of each day as a certain sort of "negotiation" where they make decisions about "how much meaning they need," where they will make that meaning, at which times they'll feel entitled to "vacations from meaning," and so on. This is a way of conceptualizing how to turn the idea of "living intentionally" into a genuine daily practice.

When you live your life as a passionate meaning-maker each day is a special sort of negotiation. You make decisions about where you will invest meaning, how you will handle activities that hold no particular meaning for you, when you will take your vacations from meaning, and so on. You make a daily bargain with yourself that if you hold to your intentions you will find no reason to doubt the meaningfulness of that day. It is like saying, "If I have a good breakfast, somehow get through the holiday buffet at the office without overdoing it, and have just one treat this evening, I won't get down on myself about what I ate today."

You do not aim for some unattainable perfection. You recognize that the three hours you spend making phone calls to nursing homes on behalf of your ailing father should definitely be toted up on the side of meaning, even if they feel like drudgery and even if the actual phoning makes you anxious. You likewise accept that you need vacations from "the whole meaning thing" on a daily basis and pencil in the novel you want to read or the movie you want to watch without the slightest bit of guilt.

Such a day may not be a "perfect" day as measured against some imaginary ideal but it is a carefully negotiated day full of hard work, service, and relaxation and a day to completely accept—and to be proud of. Your first step is to designate something as that day's primary meaning investment. If your job holds no meaning for you, that is a real problem; and you will have to decide if investing meaning in it, even though you don't receive the experience of meaningfulness in return, is the right daily meaning investment. If it isn't, you may have to treat work as "that chore" and invest daily meaning elsewhere. Whatever your job is—whether it's selling insurance, writing a novel, cleaning chimneys, or maintaining a household and a family—you will need to make daily decisions about the way you are "holding" that job.

On one day, your negotiations might sound like, "I am investing meaning in that business meeting today—I am going to go in there fully prepared and I'm going to make sure to follow up on whatever transpires—and then I'm going to take a vacation from meaning by catching up on that pile of non-essential emails waiting for me." On another day, your negotiations might sound like, "Nothing about work can be made to feel meaningful today, so I am going to invest meaning in the hour before work and in the hour after work and enjoy shopping for the crib for the new baby."

If no work tastes good to you, that is a terrible problem. If, to the description of every occupation in a manual of occupations, you respond,

"No, not particularly," that is an incipient meaning crisis. How can unhappiness not be waiting for you? Part of your daily negotiation is keeping an eye peeled for what can be experienced as meaningful, even though you have serious doubts that anything can rise to that level of its own accord. Part of the idea of investing meaning is the idea of "lifting" up work so that it rises to a place of meaningfulness.

If the work you do is a labor of love but also horribly difficult, so difficult that on most days you hate the actuality of it even as you love the idea of it, that is another genuine problem. If writing your novel or composing your symphony is pure agony, how much fun is that? How can sadness not be waiting for you? Part of your daily negotiations therefore involves reminding yourself of the meaningfulness of your work even though its execution is pure agony. This sounds like, "It is going to be pure hell getting through writing today's chapter; and whatever time I manage to spend on it will count double in my meaning calculations!"

You must also reckon with your free time. Both work time and non-work time must be accounted for in your daily negotiations. Both can be problematic: your work can feel like drudgery and your free time can feel empty. If you do not need to work, if nothing is required of you and you can just recline and count the clouds scudding by, that is its own existential problem. Have another gin and tonic? Send another text message? Recline another decade? How can sadness not be waiting for you?

Part of the negotiation process I'm describing is looking for meaning opportunities and adventures in the coming day. Say that you've been roped into going to a casino for a gambling junket and you do not care to gamble. You find yourself in a busy casino. Hundreds of people around you are playing the slot machines. You can take this as an opportunity to write a letter to your son, read a book, or do anything that you deem meaningful, even though you are stuck in the middle of a busy casino with hundreds of bells going off. Or you can just sit there bored, irritated, or furious; or, maybe even worse, gamble even though you don't care to. This junket can be a meaning opportunity—but only if you hold it that way.

Or say that you're attending a cocktail party. Party etiquette demands that you circulate and make small talk. Maybe your only goals for the evening are to survive the chatter, grab the hors d'oeuvres, and get a little tipsy. What may better serve your meaning-making needs, however, is settling in with the fellow who knows everything about the career you're contemplating starting, peppering him with questions, and maybe even asking for his help. If you feel obliged to follow party rules you may end up with another boring party experience; if you take the meaning opportunity right in front of you then you might succeed in having a meaningful experience.

All day long you make judgments and decisions, judging, for instance, that a moment has come when you had better make some meaning or else risk a meaning crisis; or deciding that plenty of meaning has been made already and that now you're entitled to a television show and some chocolate. You use your various techniques, like, for example, maintaining a morning meaning practice, reciting your life purpose statement, or touching your life purpose icon, to effectively negotiate your daily meaning challenges. These are the sorts of ideas that a meaning coach can share with clients. Over time, a meaning coach is bound to acquire all sorts of useful tactics and strategies and find his or her idiosyncratic ways of helping clients deal more effectively with their meaning challenges.

I've spent time on painting a picture of what meaning coaching looks like because I want to reinforce the idea that helping another person is not the province of only a certain class of people with titles like clinical psychologist or psychiatrist. Indeed, if you have a problem with life purpose and meaning that is causing your current despair, who would you suppose more likely to offer you relevant help, a meaning coach or a psychiatrist? A psychiatrist would have no language for communicating about these issues, no interest in exploring these issues, and would likely take you bringing them up as "symptoms of a mental disorder" and actually use them against you by adding them to some "diagnostic picture" that justified him in prescribing you chemicals. Did any of the issues I described in this chapter sound as if they would be helped by ingesting chemicals? I don't think so.

If you are just beginning to think about helping, remember that there are many ways to be of help and many kinds of helpers who can provide real, appropriate service. If you are already a helper, likewise remember that you may want to shift in one direction or another in order to make your practice more humane. To take just one example, the example I've spent time on in this chapter, you might want to shift in the direction of better understanding your clients' meaning challenges and life purpose needs. Don't you agree that those challenges and needs are almost certainly pressing and relevant? If you agree, then work to include this sort of alternative helping in your current practice.

POINTS FOR REFLECTION

1. If you haven't yet picked a professional route, what are your thoughts on becoming some sort of alternative helper rather than a traditional helper (like a psychiatrist, clinical psychologist, or psychotherapist)?

2. If you are already a working professional, what are your thoughts on adding an alternative practice (like meaning coaching) to your existing practice?

3. Do you see the need for alternative practices like meaning coaching? Do you see a place for them and a rationale for them?

4. What criteria might you use to judge whether a given alternative practice makes sense to you?

5. Is there some alternative practice that you would like to create?

16 Alternative Helping Resources for Parents, Children, and Families

Humane helping is not restricted to an office setting where one person sits across from another person. As a humane helper you might facilitate workshops, run groups, be part of a team, create a community of care, or lobby for change. You might educate readers through an informational blog or by writing books. You might start a nonprofit specializing in helping individuals plagued by a particular issue. You might bring a helping technique or point of view, for instance Finnish Open Dialogue, to the attention of sufferers unlikely to know about it. In these and in many other ways you might provide help.

Say that you wanted to help children and their parents. You could train to work one-on-one with children as a child psychologist, family therapist, or child psychiatrist. That is one path. But you might travel in a very different direction. You might create programs that you take into the schools, you might mentor youth, you might provide online resources like parenting classes or skill-building classes for teens, or in some other way provide humane help to children and their families. The routes of one-on-one talk therapy or pseudo-medical intervening are only two routes of the many that are available to you.

Consider the idea of taking informational programs into the schools. Children spend a lot of time in school. As a rule, however, schools do not see themselves as equipped to provide help with the sorts of problems that children experience. They do not see it as their responsibility or as a feature of their mandate to provide life skills classes or issue-oriented classes dealing with, for example, toxic family interactions or self-esteem and self-image issues. Some schools create peer counseling programs and in other ways try to help their students deal with their distress and difficulties, but most don't—and often simply can't.

What a school is relatively able to do, however, if its administration decides to stretch a bit, is to bring in outside programs designed to help youth with exactly these issues. These programs have many virtues. Not only is valuable information provided but it is also provided in a way that allows students to sit back in the audience and take the information in without having to react in the sort of defensive way they might in a one-on-one situation, say in a therapist's office, a psychiatrist's office, or in a heated exchange with their parents.

Consider Nicole Gibson's offerings. Nicole brings programs to schools across Australia. A finalist for Young Australian of the Year in 2014, named one of Australia's top 100 most influential women, and winner of the Pride of Australia Inspiration Medal in 2014, Nicole established The Rogue & Rouge Foundation to help Australia's young people deal with body-image issues and self-esteem issues. Taking her programs into both primary schools and high schools, she's facilitated workshops in hundreds of schools and reached hundreds of thousands of Australian youth. Her programs include nine-week well-being programs, youth motivation days, teachers' and parents' nights, a "hero within" prevention program, and more.

Nicole explained to me in an interview:

> It's important for schools to remember that they can't be everything for their students. There are valuable community organizations that specialize in the delivery of the sort of education that we do and it's the school's role to take initiative and form those crucial relationships with external organizations. Young people often tell me that it's far easier to open up to someone who's a little bit removed from their everyday world, who's closer in age and more easily relatable. For schools, it's essential to create on-going opportunities for young people to engage with this work at different ages and different intellectual and emotional levels.
>
> (Maisel, 2016b)

Isn't Nicole's an example of humane helping?

Or you might help your local schools inaugurate and run peer-counseling programs. Sande Roberts has worked in the crisis and behavioral health field for over twenty-five years and is a certified trainer of trainers in suicide prevention and crisis intervention, an advocate for peer-led programs in schools, and the author of *We Need to Talk About Suicide*. Sande explained to me in an interview:

> Peer-led teen programs have been around for a long time. Teens talk to, listen to, and believe other teens long before they consult with an adult. Schools with peer helper and conflict resolution programs have teens who are trained in peer education, leadership, listening and helping skills. The focus is on identification of problems and early intervention. My personal experience has been that teens become enabled to help themselves and their peers cope with a mega-list of relevant issues, including but not limited to suicide, violence on campus and in the community, intergenerational conflicts, relationship break-ups, dangerous relationships, scholastic pressure, and teen sexuality.
>
> (Maisel, 2016h)

Wouldn't bringing a peer-counseling program to a local school be an example of humane helping?

Then there are programs that provide mentoring, education, and community building. Consider Rob Levit's programs. Rob Levit is an award-winning creative artist and musician, nonprofit director and speaker on creativity living in Annapolis, Maryland. Rob explained to me in an interview:

> Each of our Creating Communities programs gently offers participants the opportunities to discover and engage in their own creative work. During our summer Arts Mentorship Academy, sixty youth of all ages gather for five days of intensive dance, visual art, creative writing, world drumming and singing along with mentoring and cultural enrichment activities. Here they are challenged to sit with kids they wouldn't normally choose to sit with, clean up messes they didn't make and start, and finish several projects in a week that a couple of hundred family and community members will watch on closing day.
>
> In my mind those are some good life skills to acquire! There is so much emphasis on individual achievement but when you are truly "creating communities" the life skills acquired are about trusting each

other, depending on each other and pushing each other in ways that we didn't know we were capable of. In many ways, it's an uncommon message in our current "there's an app for that" world. We ask our kids to look past "likes" and "dislikes" and find the meaning on the other side of their limits.

What kinds of outcomes and successes do we have? To take one example, last summer we had an autistic youth at the Arts Mentorship Academy. At the end of the week one of our mentors told me that the youth's guardians approached her at the final reception and asked, "What did you all do to our child?" The mentor asked, "What do you mean?" They replied, "He's actually talking to us!" They were absolutely delighted and had no idea that their own child could sing, dance, and speak on stage.

(Maisel, 2016j)

Isn't this humane helping?

Or you might provide online resources. Consider Krista MacKinnon's offerings. Krista was diagnosed with "bipolar disorder" in her formative years, never accepted the story or the drugs the system prescribed, and chose her own path to meaning, personal growth, and healing. Upon graduating from college, Krista began searching for work and found a job posting that said: "Psychiatric survivors encouraged to apply." That serendipitous event eventually led to her founding Families Healing Together, an organization that provides online classes for distressed families. Krista explained to me in an interview:

Families Healing Together helps families to understand and cope with the complicated experience of extreme distress, psychosis, and psychiatric labeling. Traditionally, when someone in a family is given a psychiatric diagnosis, families are educated to understand the experience from a brain disease/medical perspective. They often aren't given much else in terms of tools on how to heal and move forward as a family.

The philosophy of Families Healing Together is to consider all information with a critical perspective. Instead of focusing on causes, symptoms, and explanations, we propose to instead focus on deeply connected interpersonal relating, healing, and hope. We do this by sharing a curriculum filled with powerful recovery stories, helpful communication tools, and informative theories and articles about human nature. People in the class give and get support from one another as they share their personal responses to the content, and they find solace in knowing that they aren't alone in the journey.

(Maisel, 2016e)

Dan Stradford's is another sort of online resource. Dan founded the mental health nonprofit Safe Harbor in 1998 and serves as its president. He is the lead author of a guide for physicians, *Complementary and Alternative Medicine Treatments in Psychiatry*, and has published more than 250 articles and technical papers. Dan explained to me in an interview:

Safe Harbor is a nonprofit founded in 1998 by myself. Our mission is to educate the public, medical field, and government agencies on safe, non-drug treatments in mental health. Our organization coined the term "alternative mental health" because, in 1998, there was alternative medicine but no equivalent in the mental health field. We offer many articles, a bookstore, access to a self-help listserv, and a listserv for health professionals called Integrative Psychiatry. Daily we review journal articles to find recent advances in alternative mental health treatments and post the information to our listservs. Our site has now had more that 6 million visitors internationally.

(Maisel, 2016a)

There are a wide variety of organizations and services available that provide life skills and parenting education, one-to-one mentoring to youth, parent peer support, education about alternatives to chemical solutions, education about safely coming off prescribed chemicals, education about alternative approaches to handling troublesome behaviors, difficult children (for example, physically abusive children), and children suffering from anxieties and despair, hotlines and trained helpers, and workshops, classes, and often a drop-in location where parents, children, and families can receive help and support.

Consider Michael Gilbert's organization. Michael worked in human services for more than twenty-five years, including in foster care, group home, and hospital settings, and has worked for the past nineteen years as a school psychologist within the Syracuse, New York schools. In 2000, he founded It's About Childhood & Family, Inc., a not-for-profit resource center that provides families with an alternative to the traditional mental health system. Dr. Gilbert received the Friend of Children Award in 2011, the New York State Psychologist of the Year Award in 2014, and the Spirit of Huntington Award in 2014. Michael explained to me in an interview:

> Our mission at It's About Childhood & Family Inc. is to empower families to develop independence in handling life's struggles. We utilize a collaborative and trauma-informed framework that is not reliant upon a label or a diagnosis. Instead we focus on strengths, resources, resiliencies, and potential for growth. We strive to more accurately inform parents, schools, and the larger community about issues related to mental health: for example, misuse of diagnostic labels, lack of efficacy with prescription drugs, and factors that contribute to social-emotional distress.
>
> Throughout the year, we offer workshops and trainings for professionals and parents. In addition, we organize one or two conferences per year on a variety of topics such as trauma-informed care, concerns with labels and psychotropic drugs, and approaches to improve the social, emotional and behavioral well-being of children. We have brought in national and international experts in the field. Our goal is to provide a more accurate perspective and to have a dialogue about why and how to change the current mental health system, particularly for children.
>
> We encourage and provide access to a variety of approaches such as mindfulness (e.g., meditation, yoga), physical activity (e.g., running, martial arts, boxing), expressive arts (e.g., painting, pottery, photography, writing, music, dance), and relationship building (e.g., Nurtured Heart Approach, Peace Circles, Service Learning, mentoring, volunteering). In addition, we ask families to rule out potential factors that might be contributing to their problems and examine sleep patterns, nutrition, exercise, computer and television screen time, potential traumatic events, family dynamics, peer groups, educational demands, and other factors.
>
> (Maisel, 2016i)

Another approach is to identify trends and issue warnings. For example, consider the work of Sharna Olfman, who is a professor of clinical and developmental psychology at Point Park University, a psychologist in private practice, the editor/author of the Childhood in America book series for Praeger Publishers, and whose books include *The Science and Pseudoscience of Children's Mental Health: Cutting Edge Research and Treatment*, *Drugging Our Children* (coedited with Brent Robbins), *Bipolar Children*, and many others. Sharna explained to me in an interview:

> Just when it seemed that things couldn't get worse, researchers have recently noted a steep rise in the number of children who are under two years of age and being prescribed antipsychotics. Drug prescriptions for children are more often than not premised on the false assumption that they have chemical imbalances. In consequence, the real cause of their suffering, whether it be environmental or biological, goes unseen and untreated. If medication provided children with much-needed symptom relief without adverse effects then we might justify its use. Parents and children have a right to be informed about adverse long-term effects of the medications that are so readily prescribed, especially when effective therapies that do no harm are available.
>
> Along these same lines, two of the world's leading environmental scientists, Philip Landrigan and Phillipe Grandjean, have identified 1,000 neurotoxins that are either used in or are byproducts of industry that pose a direct threat to the developing brains of fetuses and young children. Several of these toxins have proven links to symptoms associated with ADHD, autism, and learning disabilities. And diets that are deficient in micronutrients (vitamins and minerals) essential for optimal brain development have also been linked to children's psychological disturbances. This research underscores the importance of healthy diet and nutritional supplements for maintaining optimal mental health. Alerting parents to these realities is one of my missions!
>
> (Maisel, 2016c)

You may already be helping in some professional capacity not directly related to mental health issues, say for example as a primary care physician or a pediatrician. As you practice and come into contact with children and their parents, it may strike you as important to help in the areas of mental and emotional help as well as in your usual ways. For instance, consider Claudia Gold. Dr. Gold, the author of *Keeping Your Child in Mind* and *The Silenced Child*, is a pediatrician who decided to turn her attention to addressing children's mental health needs from a preventative point of view. With regard to the growing practice of "screening" for so-called "mental disorders," she explained the following to me in an interview:

> If screening means the ability to identify and listen to individuals with emotional suffering, then I think it is important. But that is not what it means in our current health-care system. Screening usually involves giving a questionnaire in the primary care setting. In that setting, due in large part to our complex and powerful health insurance industry, clinicians are being forced to see more patients in less time and do not have opportunity to listen to the patient. Referral is also difficult. A severe shortage of qualified mental health professionals is integrally tied to the fact that as a culture we condone the use of psychiatric drugs in the absence of listening.
>
> This leads to the devaluing both culturally and monetarily of professionals who offer space and time for listening. In the absence of opportunity for listening, the result of screening for "mental disorders" is often the prescribing of psychiatric medication alone. We eliminate problem behavior without opportunity to discover meaning, without opportunity to learn what the behavior is communicating. In effect, we are silencing communication with this form of treatment. This is particularly worrisome in the case of postpartum depression screening where medication places the problem squarely within the mother. This approach fails to recognize the full complexity of the transition to parenthood and lets us off the hook for addressing the severe lack of social support for mothers in the postpartum period. In fact, well-meaning efforts may result in a worsening of the very problem we are trying to address by allowing us to neglect these early relationships.
>
> (Maisel, 2016k)

Maybe you're in government or the media. You can help there too. No one, including any mental health professional, has helped change Australians' minds about ADHD more than Martin Whitely. Much of Martin's focus during his twelve years as a Member of the Western

Australian Parliament went into tackling what he termed the "ADHD industry." When he was first elected in 2001 Western Australia was a world ADHD child prescribing hotspot. However, after prescribing-accountability measures were tightened in 2002, there was a 50 percent fall in Western Australia's ADHD per-capita prescribing rates by 2010. This coincided with a 51 percent fall in self-reported teenage amphetamine abuse rates in Western Australia. Martin contends this shows that if you stop giving children a free source of amphetamines they stop abusing them. He explained to me in an interview:

> Nothing demonstrates what a nonsense diagnosis ADHD is better than the now well-established late birthday effects. Four, soon to be five, large-scale international studies have established that children who are born in the later months of their school year cohort are far more likely to be labeled ADHD and drugged than their older class-mates. This late birthdate effect is just as strong in Taiwan and Western Australia where prescribing rates are relatively low as it is in North America, the home of ADHD child drugging. That says ADHD isn't over-diagnosed or overmedicated, it is fiction.
>
> Imagine if the ADHD label hadn't been invented and I suggested to you that we give amphetamines to children who frequently lose things, fidget, play too loudly, are distracted, and interrupt. You would dismiss me as either a fool or a charlatan and you would be right. The ADHD industry has been incredibly successful because they have reversed the burden of proof. Instead of them offering compelling scientific evidence that ADHD is a neurobiological disorder, the onus has been put on poorly resourced ADHD skeptics to prove it isn't.
>
> For most politicians, mental health is a mysterious field. Many believe we need to do something about mental health; however, very few have any concept of what needs to be done. As a consequence, they rely heavily on "experts" for advice. This is standard practice as politicians can't be expert in everything they are required to make decisions about. The problem is that in Australia, and I suspect internationally, most of the influential, well-resourced "experts" are industry-friendly proponents of biological psychiatry. The most dangerous of them are those that talk the language of "recovery" and "prevention" but in fact promote speculative labeling and the too-early use of biochemical interventions.

A key to changing the dominant "label and drug" paradigm is confronting the disease mongers and debunking their pseudoscience. Another key is to demand from our politicians that our regulators are independent and guided by robust science. However, it is not enough to just win the debate in the scientific literature. It needs to be won in the media, both social and traditional. So much of the excesses of biological psychiatry like ADHD and juvenile bipolar disorder are ripe for ridicule. If you can win the popular culture debate, public opinion and therefore our political leaders will follow.

(Maisel, 2016g)

Maybe you're a lawyer. Consider the important work done by Jim Gottstein. Jim is a lawyer in private practice in Anchorage, Alaska, whose Law Project for Psychiatric Rights is a public interest law firm devoted to the defense of people facing forced psychiatric drugging and electroshock. Jim explained to me:

PsychRights' mission is to mount a strategic litigation campaign against forced psychiatric drugging and electroshock. In Alaska, PsychRights has won five Alaska Supreme Court cases (and lost a couple). The Alaska Supreme Court has held in PsychRights cases that the government cannot drug someone against their will unless it can prove by clear and convincing evidence that it is in the person's best interest and there is no less intrusive alternative available.

As terrible as the psychiatric drugging and electroshocking of adults is, the drugging of children is even more horrific. I have a hard time coming up with an adjective strong enough for the carnage caused by the widespread psychiatric drugging of children, especially poor children on Medicaid. This is an unfolding national tragedy of immense proportions, the results of which we don't even know yet.

Poor children are so vulnerable because their parents don't have the social standing to resist schools and child protective services insisting their children be drugged to suppress behavior that disturbs the adults. Despite laws to the contrary, parents are told their children will be thrown out of school if they are not given the drugs and often threatened with having their children taken from them on the grounds that the parents are neglecting the child's medical need to be drugged.

Both of these threats are often carried out. God help foster children because they are particularly at the mercy of bureaucrats who have been brainwashed by Big Pharma to drug children.

(Maisel, 2016d)

You might even create a tour! Marilyn Wedge is a family therapist and the author of three books, most recently *A Disease called Childhood: Why ADHD Became an American Epidemic*. Dr. Wedge holds a doctorate from the University of Chicago, was a post-doctoral fellow at the Hastings Center for Bioethics, and is the creator of the Reclaiming Childhood tour. Marilyn explained to me in an interview:

The Reclaiming Childhood tour is a series of one day seminars across the country led by experts in a variety of fields—school counseling, psychology, medical journalism, research, and family therapy. We intend to spark a much-needed discussion regarding children's mental health and well-being.

Our society's perception of childhood has undergone a dramatic change in the last four decades. Behaviors that were previously considered a part of normal childhood, a child's normal reaction to stress in their social environment, or normal developmental phases have been redefined as 'mental disorders' that require treatment with psychiatric drugs. Children are being medicated with anti-depressants and anti-psychotics that were not FDA-approved for children and which have dangerous side effects. Even stimulant drugs typically prescribed for ADHD are proving to have dangerous side effects like psychotic episodes.

Based on our many years of research and experience, the speakers on the Reclaiming Childhood tour offer a new paradigm of child mental health informed by the latest research in neuroscience as well as many years of clinical experience with children. We offer safe, effective solutions for childhood difficulties—family therapy, parenting classes, school interventions, dietary interventions, and a host of others. As we speak around the country to parents, educators, and therapists, we expect to ignite a tipping point in the way our society perceives the difficulties and challenges of childhood and how we can best help children at home and at school.

(Maisel, 2016f)

Whether you have a desire to help children or to help adults, there are many ways that you can prove of help. The "office" model, where a helper sits with an individual and "diagnoses and treats" or "engages in psychotherapy," is only one model. You might start a website, start a nonprofit, become an advocate or an activist, work in a team or group setting, prepare programs that you deliver to particular audiences, mentor youths or adults, write and educate, or use your current expertise as a lawyer, physician, academic, researcher, journalist, or other working professional in the service of helping individuals with their mental health concerns. Humane helping doesn't come in one size or shape and all of its many sizes and shapes are needed.

POINTS FOR REFLECTION

1. Is there some program that you would like to create and deliver?

2. Is there an online resource that you would like to create and manage?

3. Is there a nonprofit or other organization that you would like to create and build?

4. Are there some classes or workshops that you would like to create and facilitate?

5. Is there some alternative way of delivering humane helping that might particularly suit you?

REFERENCES

Maisel, E. (2016a). "Day 2: Dan Stradford on Safe Harbor and Mental Health Change." *Psychology Today*. www.psychologytoday.com/blog/rethinking-mental-health/201601/day-2-dan-stradford-safe-harbor-and-mental-health-change
Maisel, E. (2016b). "Day 3: Nicole Gibson & Australia's Rogue & Rouge Foundation." *Psychology Today*. www.psychologytoday.com/blog/rethinking-mental-health/201601/day-3-nicole-gibson-australias-rogue-rouge-foundation

Maisel, E. (2016c). "Day 9: Sharna Olfman on Child Mental Health Controversies." *Psychology Today*. www.psychologytoday.com/blog/rethinking-mental-health/201601/day-9-sharna-olfman-child-mental-health-controversies

Maisel, E. (2016d). "James Gottstein on Psychiatry and Your Legal Rights." *Psychology Today*. www.psychologytoday.com/blog/rethinking-mental-health/201605/james-gottstein-psychiatry-and-your-legal-rights

Maisel, E. (2016e). "Krista MacKinnon on Families Healing Together." *Psychology Today*. www.psychologytoday.com/blog/rethinking-mental-health/201602/krista-mackinnon-families-healing-together

Maisel, E. (2016f). "Marilyn Wedge on Reclaiming Childhood." *Psychology Today*. www.psychologytoday.com/blog/rethinking-mental-health/201603/marilyn-wedge-reclaiming-childhood

Maisel, E. (2016g). "Martin Whitely on ADHD" *Psychology Today*. www.psychologytoday.com/blog/rethinking-mental-health/201603/martin-whitely-adhd

Maisel, E. (2016h). "Mentoring Kids in Distress: An Interview with Sande Roberts." *Psychology Today*. www.psychologytoday.com/blog/rethinking-mental-health/201701/mentoring-kids-in-distress

Maisel, E. (2016i). "Michael Gilbert on It's About Childhood and Family, Inc." *Psychology Today*. www.psychologytoday.com/blog/rethinking-mental-health/201604/michael-gilbert-its-about-childhood-and-family-inc

Maisel, E. (2016j). "Rob Levit on Mentoring and Creating Communities." *Psychology Today*. www.psychologytoday.com/blog/rethinking-mental-health/201602/rob-levit-mentoring-and-creating-communities

Maisel, E. (2016k). "The Silenced Child: An Interview with Claudia Gold." *Psychology Today*. www.psychologytoday.com/blog/rethinking-mental-health/201612/the-silenced-child

17 Shifting Your Practices

A humane helper ought to look at her current practices and honestly decide what portion of what she is doing is the right and appropriate thing to do, what portion she is doing because it is the customary and accepted thing to do (like providing labels that then stick for life), what portion she is doing for her own ego, so that she can feel like an expert and a professional, and what portion she is doing simply to get paid, for example via insurance reimbursement.

After she has teased this all apart she may decide that there are certain changes that she would like to make in her practices. She might, for example, create a new intake form that does a fuller job of inquiring into a client's current circumstances, goals, and aspirations. She might stop calling the people she sees "patients" (in keeping with distancing herself from anything pseudo-medical sounding). She might adopt a very ordinary vocabulary that includes words like sadness, disappointment, frustration, resentment, and grievance. She might educate herself about alternative resources like mentoring and peer counseling resources, psychiatric survivor networks, and so on.

If you're in private practice, not reliant on insurance reimbursement or government health plans, and have a broad mandate as a feature of your license or certification, you can more easily make any shifts you deem desirable. But what if you find yourself inside an organization, institution, or system that limits your ability to be yourself, that operates from the pseudo-medical labeling model, and that demands that you follow specific procedures and specific treatment plans? What then?

Let's picture a helper we'll call Mary who works as a psychologist at a HMO and whose duties include running psychotherapy groups, doing individual psychotherapy, administering psychological tests, serving on assessment and treatment teams, and supervising interns. In what ways might Mary shift her practices so as to humanize her helping? Here are several efforts she might make:

She might refresh her memory as to the basis of psychological testing and see which, if any, of the psychological tests she currently administers she still believes in. She might remind herself that test reliability is a less important matter than test validity: what's most important is whether or not a given test actually makes sense.

For example, given the precise way that a test like the Minnesota Multiphasic Personality Inventory (MMPI) was normed, by identifying question responses that distinguished institutionalized "mental patients" from non-mental patients, and given what we now know about how often people found (and find) themselves in mental hospitals for completely non-medical reasons, is the MMPI really a valid instrument? As she refreshes her memory in this way, she may discover that certain tests that she routinely administers ought to be jettisoned.

And what if her HMO won't allow such independent decision-making or independent action? Then she must decide to what extent she wants to be an activist (and perhaps jeopardize her career). She might opt for high activism and lobby within the HMO for major changes or she might opt for low activism and see if there is some way to quietly test less or quietly switch to more valid tests.

She might raise her voice—quietly or more loudly—in assessment and treatment planning meetings and lobby for less quick labeling, less pseudo-medical posturing, and less chemical intervening. If this means that she ends up butting heads with a given psychiatrist or a given team administrator, it will mean precisely that. Every committee has its personalities, its cliques, and its divided opinions; and, if she is willing, she can join her committee's "critical" camp or stand alone as the voice of dissent. She might raise her voice aggressively or rather more quietly, depending in part on her personality and in part on how much she wants to safeguard her job.

When supervising her interns, she might suggest that they do the radical thing of reading up in the critical psychology, critical psychiatry, and antipsychiatry literature rather than accepting the two dominant paradigms—the pseudo-medical one and the expert talk one—without scrutiny. If she needs to buttress her contention that scrutiny is good, she might point her interns to the article in the *Schizophrenia Bulletin* written by the psychiatrist Sir Robin Murray (2016) in which he confesses, "If I had the chance to have a second career, I would try harder not to follow the fashion of the herd. The mistakes I have made, at least those into which I have insight, have usually resulted from adhering excessively to the prevailing orthodoxy."

She might likewise suggest that, rather than trying to figure out what label to provide for the clients that they see, that her interns spend a great deal of time leaning forward, being curious, and experiencing the full humanness of the human beings sitting across from them. She might suggest that they do this even if that makes them more anxious than programmatically knowing what to do next and even if that is harder work than consulting a checklist and providing a label.

She might regularly ask her interns, "What would your client like to try?" rather than "What would you like to try?", she might ask them, "What game plan have the two of you created?" rather than "What's your treatment plan?" and in these and other ways underline that psychotherapy means forging relationships and taking the expressed concerns and desires of clients into account.

In the groups that she runs she might steer participants away from self-identifying as patients, as ill, as mentally disordered, as "having something" ("I have PTSD" or "I have a learning disability"), or as "being something" ("I'm bipolar" or "I'm ADD") and toward the idea that life is challenging, that there are insights they can gain and valuable coping skills and new habits they can learn, and that their life is a project that requires their involvement and attention.

Likewise, she might create measured language to use that allows her to explain her beliefs about the chemicals participants may be taking without putting herself at odds with her institution. This latter task is immensely tricky—but nevertheless an important part of the shift she is endeavoring to make away from the current pseudo-medical model.

Whether, like Mary, you find yourself inside a constricting institution, whether you are in private practice but still constrained by your license to operate in certain ways, or whether you are in an unregulated helping profession like coaching, the following nine shifts will help you move in the direction of providing humane care that matches your updated understanding of what helps to reduce emotional suffering and mental distress:

1. The first shift is a shift in the direction of clarity and honesty. Get clear on what you are currently doing. What is actually going on between you and the people you see? Is the bulk of that nothing fancier than "chatting about life problems"? If it is, do you nevertheless rather automatically place such ordinary helpful conversations in the context of the "diagnosing and treating mental disorders" paradigm for no other reason than that is what you have been taught to do or are accustomed to doing?

What medical-looking activities actually go on in session? If the answer is none, then think through how you might honor the good work you are doing while at the same time dropping the habit of "diagnosing and treating mental disorders." This may prove to be more like an earthquake than a simple shift but it is important and honorable work.

2. Make the shift in your own mind from "mental disease thinking" to "problems in living thinking." Rather than automatically ticking off squirming as a "symptom" of the "mental disorder of ADHD" or gloominess as a "symptom" of the "mental disorder of clinical depression," train yourself to ask yourself the question, "I wonder why little Johnny is squirming?" or "I wonder why Jane is gloomy?"

Learn to lead with "I wonder what's going on?" rather than with "What mental disorder can I detect?" Stop looking for mental disorders just because shopping catalogues for mental disorders, the DSM and the ICD, happen to exist and happen to have been foisted upon you. This may not prove a shift that you can accomplish easily or accomplish overnight, especially if your interactions with colleagues, HMOs, and even friends and family pull at you to retain a "disorder label" way of talking.

3. Make the shift from "I need to look like an expert" to "I need to be human." You entered a helping profession for many reasons but among them was the desire to look like an expert, to be accorded the material and psychological perks that professionals receive, and to have your ego massaged by being called "doctor" or "counselor" or something similar. Now it is time to be a human being again.

It is lovely to feel associated with medical doctors as a "doctor of the mind" and it is of course appropriate to be paid like a professional for the work that you do. But isn't the work that you do rather like the work that anyone with human experience skills and some wisdom about life also does? Isn't it what a sponsor in AA does, what a peer counselor in a high school does, what a wise aunt does, or what anyone who understands life, who listens and who responds appropriately does?

It isn't that you need to apologize for the fact that you aren't doing "real medicine" or announce that you aren't really a professional. Rather this shift is internal, away from acting like you have the answers (which is the stance we want from our plumber, lawyer, or accountant) and toward the attitude of an experimentalist, one who, like any scientist, has tools, tactics, and ideas but who, for example, doesn't really know what transpired before the big bang occurred until he really does know. A plumber fixes and a scientist asks questions. You can still be the professional you want to be: just shift away from plumber and toward scientist.

SHIFTING FROM THE BIOMEDICAL TO THE TRANSPERSONAL: ONE VIEW

Katie Mottram is a founding director of the International Spiritual Emergence Network and the author of *Mend the Gap: A Transformative Journey from Deep Despair to Spiritual Awakening*. She explained to me:[1]

Let's compare the outcomes of two different approaches to the same problem, the approach of the dominant biomedical paradigm versus the approach of an alternative transpersonal paradigm.

Take two people who have had similar trauma in early childhood: the loss of their mother in their formative years. They grew up in families where death was not openly discussed, and so repressed their grief, trying to "be strong" for the sake of their father and siblings. Both develop depression and anxiety in adolescence and start drinking to mask their pain, causing mood swings. Both have strived for happiness to overcome this hidden pain in achievements and in lives that appear "successful" to society; they are sociable at times and at other times feel lost and isolated. Both come to the attention of mental health services when they attempt suicide at the age of thirty.

Now their paths diverge:

Client A is seen by a psychiatrist, one who has learned and practices the reductionist, biomedical model of pathologizing presenting symptoms. She is diagnosed with bipolar disorder, put on a mood-stabilizing drug, and told she'll likely need it for life, given that she has a mental disorder. Her sense of self-confidence plummets further, she feels ashamed, she puts on weight due to the drugs, and she goes on to lose her job due to a lack of motivation. Her drinking increases in an effort to further mask the sense of worthlessness and shame she feels at having a "mental illness" that she has been told she has no control over.

Client B is seen by a transpersonal psychotherapist who explores the reasons behind the suicide attempt, investigating the history and feelings of client B prior to her suicide attempt. Time is taken to develop a safe space to talk and to investigate the emotions that she's been repressing for years. Her emotions are normalized and she is supported in processing them, allowing the grief to surface and be released. Accordingly, she feels a sense of trust and is able to discuss death in a way that was never possible at the time of her mother's passing. She gradually feels able to open up further about her "anomalous" experiences, namely the sense that she has received communication from her deceased mother since her mother's passing.

She is given information to normalize this experience, transpersonal guidance to assist her growth, and encouraged to learn to discern what might be her own intuition about these experiences. As a result, she acquires a stronger sense of self and self-compassion and begins to feels the most authentic she has ever felt. She continues to flourish and goes on to work at a job that brings her personal joy, rather than worrying about external achievements.

The most important difference between these two scenarios is the second therapist's ability to be "human" herself, in touch with her own emotions, knowledgeable about her own triggers, and able to be compassionate toward herself and therefore toward others. The psychiatrist working with Client A operates from a detached hierarchical perspective whereas the trans-personal psychotherapist works alongside Client B to encourage personal growth, believing that she is going through a difficult but essentially positive transformation process.

4. Fourth, shift your actual tactics, strategies, and practices. Think through what changes you intend to make in the way you interact with the people you see. Do you want to stop calling them "patients" and stop pretending that you are doing medicine? Do you want to ask different questions in session, respond in different ways, or propose more experiments? If you would like to become more of a humane helper, what would that look like in session?

That new, different look might take countless concrete forms. You might begin to role-play and rehearse upcoming situations in session, for example in order to help a shy person get ready for a job interview or to prepare a beleaguered wife to speak up for her rights. You might wonder aloud about what might be causing a sufferer's sadness, using a very ordinary vocabulary that includes words like disappointment, frustration, resentment, grievance, and so on. You might present information, say about available community resources or stress-management techniques, even if that feels more like social work, consulting, coaching, or teaching than psychotherapy.

5. Fifth is a shift toward a deep acceptance of the fact that you don't really know what's going on in and with the person sitting across from you. It is good to become much easier with that not knowing (as we discussed earlier). Admit out loud that you don't know; that the two of you are guessing; that your suggestions are more like experiments that may prove fruitful than like expert advice that comes with guarantees.

At the same time remember that all this not knowing doesn't mean that you can't have ideas about what might help and tactics and strategies for helping. We may not know what is causing a fire but in the absence of counter-indications we think that throwing water on it makes sense. We may not know what is causing our shortness of breath but in the absence of counter-indications we think that sitting down and resting make sense.

We act but we also appraise: we throw water on the fire but we register if the fire flares up; we catch our breath but we also register that our chest feels uncharacteristically tight and that we had better dial 911. The same is true with respect to helping someone in distress. As we work with sufferers we both act and appraise. We are able to act because we have a sense of what to do even if we don't know the exact chain of cause and effect affecting our client. Our abundant not knowing doesn't prevent us from being useful and helpful.

6. Sixth is a shift in the direction of paying much more attention than you may currently be doing to the role of socioeconomic conditions and other social and cultural realities in the lives of the sufferers you see (as discussed previously). That poor people, marginalized people, children in foster care, and other human beings who are struggling and who are at the mercy of the power structure receive mental disorder labels at a far higher rate than do their more privileged brothers and sisters should alert you to the sociocultural components of distress, difficulty, suffering, acting out and top-down mental disorder labeling.

You will want to better understand the power of society to inflict emotional distress and exert control, as for instance when it labels a person for life with one or another mental disorder label. You will want to not forget that "diagnosing and treating mental disorders" is a societal game. In one edition, the DSM designates homosexuality a mental disorder; in another it doesn't: that isn't medicine but the power structure making top-down decisions about what is "normal" and what is "abnormal." All of this you will keep in mind.

7. Another valuable shift you'll want to contemplate making is a shift in the direction of advocating for a mental wellness movement that includes better conditions for everyone, less poverty, less hunger, less ignorance, less cruelty, more love—fewer of the bad things and more of the good things.

You might advocate for mental wellness and societal change in staff meetings, in blog posts, and in conversations with your colleagues and shift boldly in the direction of advocacy. You might pick a particular hobbyhorse and, for example, lobby for the teaching of life skills in elementary school, the creation of more communities of care, or the provision of public service announcements that caution against the current ubiquitous chemical fix for emotional distress. Your mantra might become, "I demand more of myself and I demand more of the system."

8. You might also need to shift in the direction of not flinching in the face of pushback to your advocacy and criticism of your new positions. One of the features of our species is that smart folks who do not want to tell the truth, perhaps because they have a financial interest in not telling the truth, can argue smartly against whatever a truth-teller is saying, and embroil him in a time-consuming game where he feels obliged to answer each and every one of their objections. When these carefully crafted distortions of your position and loud objections start to come at you—about what a dangerous game you're playing by "preventing schizophrenics from getting the medication they need" or by "planting seeds of doubt about the helping professions"—try not to flinch.

Be prepared for this pushback. Your colleagues may well disagree with your position, feel the need to voice their disagreement, and even break with you now that you are in the "enemy camp." Some of these breaks you may welcome and others may cause you genuine pain. A necessary shift to accompany your movement to your new position as an at least occasional naysayer and whistle blower is a shift in the direction of invulnerability to pushback.

Offer your new proposals, argue for your vision of a different future, and say what you think is true, including fearlessly acknowledging all that isn't known and all that maybe never will be known. Rather than flinch in the face of objections or spend a lot of time arguing with opponents, stand straighter and fight harder.

9. An important shift is getting clear on the difference between a "difficult person" and a "mentally diseased person," as discussed previously. A humane helper does not start from the place that "human beings are born to be happy and any deviation from 'happy' is abnormal and a mental disorder." Instead, she starts from the following place, not so different

from the place where a Buddhist starts: "Life is difficult and produces many challenges and sources of pain, confusion, and despair; all this pain, confusion and despair are of course unwanted but natural enough and should not be 'diagnosed' away or minimized away."

That she honors all this doesn't mean that she shakes her head and murmurs, "Ah, well, too bad." She fervently wants the person sitting across from her to suffer less, to feel less emotional pain, to do less harm to himself (and to others), and to feel happier and more inclined to go on living. His pain, darkness, and difficulty are natural—but that is not to say that they are acceptable, immutable, or incontrovertible. She works to reduce all that: but her starting point is to nod and announce, as she does again and again in her work with struggling mortals, "How very human."

The number of shifts required to move from the expert/pseudo-medical model to the humane helper model—from the white-coat model to the collaborative model—are many, more than just the nine I've described above. You will want to shift in the direction of familiarizing yourself with the experiences of sufferers, service users, and the psychiatric survivor movement (as discussed previously). You will want to shift in the direction of paying a lot of attention to life purpose issues and meaning challenges in the lives of your clients (as discussed previously). But the primary shift, however, and the one that takes all other shifts into account is the basic shift in paradigm: shifting to the paradigm of humane helping.

The phrase "paradigm shift" is used rather frequently and loosely to provide added luster to a speaker's preferred way of thinking. Here, I think, it is justified. When you stop believing that the laundry list of mental disorders that currently exists and the chemical dispensing that flows from that aberrant list-making are either right or proper and instead start believing that your job isn't to "diagnose and treat mental disorders" but to be there for another human being and help relieve him of his often-severe human distress, that is nothing less than a radical paradigm shift in your way of thinking.

It is the radical shift from looking for assorted leaks in the plumbing to acknowledging that life is difficult. That is the primary shift required of you. It certainly isn't the case that current working professionals—clinical psychologists, family therapists, clinical social workers, psychiatrists, psychotherapists, etc.—have no place in an improved, more human, and humane mental health system. But I do believe that current working professionals are obliged to rethink their model and their practices, shift from "mental disease thinking" to "problems in living thinking," and become more humane in practice.

This fundamental shift involves a repudiation of the DSM (and, where applicable, the ICD). It involves a repudiation of the idea that "collections of symptoms" are entitled to be called by made-up, medical-sounding labels. It involves a repudiation of the idea that without some real investigating we know what, other than ordinary life, is causing a boy to squirm or a girl to be sad. It involves a repudiation of the idea that we can ever really know what is causing human reactions like anxiety or sadness and a simultaneous embracing of our ability to be of help even if we don't know. It especially involves a repudiation of the idea that some form of medicine is going on. This movement away from prescription pads and made-up labels and toward honesty and clarity is comprised of the sorts of shifts, efforts, and initiatives I've described above. I hope you'll join me and embrace the paradigm of humane helping.

POINTS FOR REFLECTION

1. Describe the ways in which you might shift your practice in the direction of more humane helping.

2. If those shifts are likely to produce pushback and criticism, how will you deal with that pushback and criticism?

3. Which shifts feel like they would be easy to make and which feel like they would be hard?

4. What are your concluding ideas about what humane helping means?

5. What are your thoughts about how you might become a more humane helper?

NOTE

1 In private correspondence.

REFERENCE

Murray, R. M. (2016). "Mistakes I Have Made in My Research Career," *Schizophrenia Bulletin*, December 21. https://academic.oup.com/schizophrenia bulletin/article-abstract/43/2/253/2730504/Mistakes-I-Have-Made-in-My-Research-Career?redirectedFrom=PDF

Index

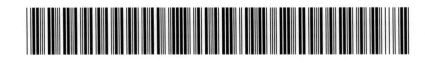